Angel Kisses
No More Cancer

An Emotional Journey of
Love, Loss, Courage, and Hope

Stacie Overman
Founder of the New You Program

Edited by Qat Wanders, Jean Pace, and Jaime Lea of Wandering Words Media

Proofread by Dee Turner

Cover design by Heidi Sutherlin

Please visit

www.stacieoverman.com/gift

for your free gift!

Dedication

To my dear husband, Larry.

To my amazing father and mother, Jim and Viki, for always being there for me.

*To my daughter, Alex—
may you see the greatness within you.*

To all the Earth Angels, may you find the New You waiting inside to be released and shine your light so brightly.

Acknowledgments

To my dear husband, Larry, for helping to make it possible for me to share my journey with the world. Encouraging me to complete the book and holding space for me to be my best.

To my dear momma, for always being there for me, heart to heart.

To Qat, my patient editor. Thank you for bearing with me in my learning curve of completing a book and your support and understanding of working with an Angel Channeler.

To my beautiful Host of Angels that lovingly chuckle at my learning curve of being a soul having a human experience. They have given me such peace, love, and joy and have taught me how to share the Christ Consciousness with the world.

And most of all, I give the utmost gratitude to God, for always being with me even when I was wrestling in the depths of despair. Thank you for always showing me the light and love in all situations. Thank for having patience with me while I found myself so I then could shine my light so brightly. Thank you for impressing it upon my heart to help profoundly change the lives of thousands of beautiful souls. By helping them heal on a mind, body and soul level so they can find the light within themselves.

Praise for

Angel Kisses

No More Cancer

"Stacie Overman's incredible story of a family facing and overcoming cancer inspired me to see my own life with a fresh perspective and humble appreciation. With empathy, she conveys beautiful higher truths learned – in a way that is grounded in reality – including some of the gritty "nuts and bolts" of the experiences. Not insignificantly, the book is a beautiful celebration of Stacie's second husband, Hank, which I am thankful for."

~ Andrea Schmidt,
A-Schmidt Graphic Design & Abstract Art

"Stacie has opened my mind and heart to the idea of Angels. This book is an amazing story that shows the journey of a truly inspirational spiritual teacher."

~Racheal Richard,
Breast Cancer Survivor / New You Program Graduate

"Angel Kisses is a pivotal book in helping others understand the power of their connection. Stacie's amazing and beautiful connection with the angels and beyond is not only inspiring but empowering. Her courage to believe and have faith shows everyone what is possible.

Stacie's trust in her guidance, even when she didn't recognize it, proves to me we are always being held in the loving arms of Source. I for one am so happy this tenacious lady overcame the odds and chose to use her voice to show others what is possible. Thank you for trusting and sharing."

Much Love and Peace,

~ Liza Jane Wolf,
Psychic Medium and Spiritual Teacher

"Stacie's story is one of triumph and tragedy and will resonate with anyone who has been touched by cancer. She weaves a love story for the ages with a bittersweet conclusion into her own cancer journey. This book illustrates her triumph in summoning the powerful energy of the Source of all creation to enact miracles while guiding her husband through his journey with a different but no less powerful outcome.

I highly recommend *Angel Kisses*, it will guide and enlighten and illuminate that each

journey is different and there is expansion in every outcome."

~David Strickel
Channel of The Stream
Author of *The Stream - Eternal Wisdom For a Better Life*
Host of The Stream of David Show & podcast

"I was an awakened being since early childhood; however, I blocked my gifts due to fear. Since I've met Stacie Overman, a Divine spiritual master, I was always fearful; now, by being a member of her group and her support, I am ready to discover my soul purpose."

-Leslie Elizabeth,
member of Understanding Divine Messages

"I've experienced firsthand how God uses specific soul connections to catalyze change and awaken gifts. When one reads Stacie's story, such a divinely orchestrated shift in paths is obvious!"

-Kerry McQuisten,
Publisher, Black Lyon Publishing, LLC

"In 1998, I lost my beloved Judi after a valiant three year odyssey with cancer. It was a time of discovery, deep faith, and personal insights for both of us. Stacie Overman's *Angel Kisses No More Cancer* brought tears to my eyes as she shared the "grace and grit" of her personal battle with cancer and the loss of her partner, Hank. Her story of love, loss, courage, healing, and inspiration is one that our world needs and needs now! Thank you, Stacie."

-Victor Fuhrman,
Host and Producer, OmTimes Destination Unlimited

Here is to God's will being done and Archangel Gabriel's beautiful energy filling you and me.

Contents

Foreword

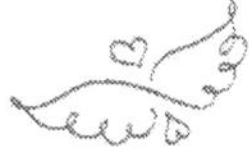

Some will say angels come in many forms, in a variety of ways, and they will come to us during our darkest of hours as well as celebrate with us in our happiest of moments.

I believe that all angels are of and from God, and it is He who oversees all of Earth's blessed beings, and coordinates this extremely delicate dance that we call life. All the while, God is balancing each soul's encounter, coordinating our intertwining journeys, and bringing His glorious angels in, through, and around our lives to help all of us to see and experience His love.

For me, Stacie, coming into my life was what I like to refer to as Divine intervention. It was God bringing a human angel into my world, one who would show and remind me that despite all of the hardships, heartache, pain, and disappointments, that love from God would help to bring me back to my true self. I knew Stacie was a gift to me, God's way of putting this genuine, loving, beautiful and determined soul—His earth angel—right into my path. This helped me recapture my heart song and led me back to my true self.

At the time I met Stacie, my soul, my heart song was really having a very hard time singing. Life's trials and tribulations, along with several ongoing heartbreaks had negatively impacted me and my heart song was getting lost. And then this earth angel, Stacie Overman, came along!

My first phone call with Stacie will be forever etched in my mind. I couldn't figure out if it was real, or if I was only imagining this incredible conversation with this beautiful, God-filled and loving person, who felt like my best friend during that first conversation. Was this just wishful thinking or could I really trust this person and my feelings? It became quite obvious, rather quickly, that God had arranged our meeting and its purpose had been preplanned. It was a moment of gentle clarity, when we had a shared vision, a message—one which brought both laughter and heartfelt tears to both of us. It was a clear sign that God was definitely at work and was in charge of the meaning behind it all.

Through Stacie, I came to a deep sense of safety and a feeling of genuine hope. This was something I had not felt in a very long time. God had sent me a true soul friend, His earth angel, and it was like getting a warm, love-filled hug from Him, with a side of gentle Angel kisses! I'm forever grateful to Him, and to Stacie, for their unconditional love!

Through Stacie's incredibly special friendship, her true belief in me and who I am, along with the needed healing and inner growth that I gained from her beautiful program, I found my way back to myself. I healed my broken spirit and learned so much more about who I really am. I am embracing the unique and special gifts that God has given to me, and I am working on sharing them so much more now. Stacie helped me hear the angelic voices I needed to hear to bring me comfort and guidance, and now I can channel the voices of the angels myself. I'm even singing and sharing my heart song again! Meeting Stacie is something I now consider one of the biggest God/soul-checks of my lifetime! How precious to be able to say I found not only myself and my heart song again, but also a best friend and a soul sister. All of it because of God's love and His plan.

And for you, all those who will be reading Stacie's story, sharing in her journey and lessons in strength and love, may each of you receive what you may need to help your own heart song and soul to sing!

Many blessings and love,

Debbie Motyka

About This Book

Why I Do What I Do

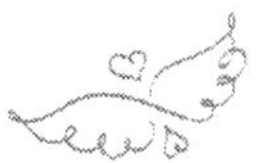

In the following pages, I am about to share with you a deep part of myself. I am going to let you have a peek at my soul. There is a lot more to this story than just my journey with cancer. Everything changed after that. I mean everything. I am not the same person I was before. I mean that on so many levels—physical, emotional, spiritual. Especially spiritual. I am a whole new me.

Okay, I will just come right out and say it: coming so close to death brought me closer to my angels. I can communicate with them in ways I never before dreamed were possible. They speak to me and through me now. I see them. I hear them. I feel them.

The best part is that I am now able to share these messages with you, too. Sometimes their messages just come through so strong I can't help but want to share them with the world! That is part of why this book came to be. It's also a big part of why I started my New You Program, but we will get to that later. Interspersed throughout my story, you will be able to read some of the direct communications I had with angels. I included one at the end of each chapter. Angels speak to me and, through this book, they can speak to you. They are dictated at the end of each chapter exactly as they came to me. I hope you can find comfort in their words, as I have.

For now, sit back and get comfy. Grab a cup of tea and prop up your feet. Not only am I going to invite you to follow along with me on this beautiful journey where you are more than welcome to laugh and cry along with me, but I am also going to share messages with you directly from my angel guides. So many of them have stepped forward to share messages that I am so excited to pass along to you! So take a deep breath and get ready. I'm going to tell you my story . . .

Preface

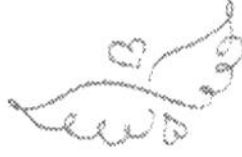

"They told me I'm dying." I said the words to my mom over the phone.

This was after my second chemo treatment. I got it every other Friday and my husband got chemo opposite me, also every other Friday. I was home alone, lying in bed in my three-story house with my cordless phone pressed against my face. Mom had called, but I had no energy. I couldn't even hold the receiver, so it was propped up next to me. Yesterday, when they told me I was dying, I didn't feel like I was.

"But today I feel like I am," I told my mother in a pain-filled voice. As I was speaking, I could feel every bone in my body aching, especially my sternum. I was lying on my pillow with tears streaming out of my eyes and rolling down my cheeks. I could feel her wanting to be with me, but she was in another state. I knew she just wanted to hold her baby, and I just wanted my mommy.

My husband was also battling cancer at that time and there were times neither of us could go down the nineteen stairs, so we had a mini fridge and surround sound in the room. It was an old house that my husband had rebuilt and renovated. It had a big archway to see into the bathroom which had a garden tub.

As I was lying on the bed, I looked in the bathroom and wondered if I could even make it there. There was a rocker recliner next to the bed, and I didn't even have the strength to get to the chair. I couldn't turn on the television because all the sound did was hurt my body.

There were two windows in the room, I could look out to see the birds and the tall pine trees. The view was absolutely beautiful. But because I was lying there so much, my husband was worried my chemo would settle in my bladder and burn a hole there, so he got a huge mason jar, set it next to my bed, and said, "I want you to drink this whole thing."

I was never a big water drinker but now, with chemo, it tasted like a ground-up penny on my tongue. I couldn't drink more than two sips all day.

This memory is forever etched in my mind. I can still hear the birds chirping outside the window. I can smell the earthy scent of the pine trees wafting in with the gentle breeze. As I write this, it tastes as if the metallic flavor lingers on my tongue, and I press my hand to my heart as I recall the pain in my chest. Tears fill my eyes even now. They told me I'm dying.

Chapter One

The Fight for the New Me

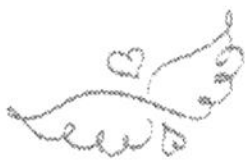

Fourteen years ago, I heard the words, "You have cancer." Hopefully, in October, I'll be able to say I'm twelve years in remission. I'm a 49-year-old breast cancer survivor, a mom, and I lost my soulmate about eight years ago to a rare form of cancer. I went to work for the American Cancer Society shortly after he passed away. I was a community relations manager, and I helped to put on three Relay for Life events within three different communities in Oregon, raising funds to find a cure for cancer. After several years, I realized I needed to focus on building a spiritual community of thriving survivors in my New You Program. I am, and continue to be, an advocate for finding a cure for cancer and being a voice for survivors and caregivers everywhere. I know my purpose is to help others in their own health struggles like an "earth angel."

An earth angel is someone who comes to Earth to help others through a specific struggle. I believe we go through certain life events so we can help others through the same. I am grateful I was able to help people with cancer through my work with the American Cancer Society. Through our struggle, we become a light to help others. And I look forward to helping people in their spiritual journey through my New You Program as well.

I am very passionate about helping other people and being a source of motivation and inspiration to others. I was 36 years old when I was diagnosed with breast cancer. The doctors told me if I hadn't found it when I did, I wouldn't have lived for three more years. So I wouldn't have made my 40th birthday or experienced the birth of my first grandchild.

At the time, my children were seven, eight, and 15. The scariest part of being diagnosed with cancer was wondering what was going to happen—the unknown. How bad was it going to be? Was it going to hurt? Would I be sick? Everyone is different, and it was impossible to know what my exact symptoms would be.

I laid in bed every night thinking about how this would affect my children. I was so terrified of not being able to comfort them. Or to not to be able to be there for them in my physical form. The scariest part was wondering if they would be okay without me. Every mom knows the most terrifying thing is to not be there for your child in his/her time of need. My mind raced, creating different scenarios where I would not be able to be there for them.

I was so fortunate to have such great resources right in my own community. I was blessed that I didn't have to drive a couple of hours away to Portland, Oregon, and could stay in my hometown of Eugene. If I'd had to travel, it would have been difficult to take enough time off of work and the cost of traveling would have been a difficult expense. For us, since my husband was also having chemo treatments, these struggles would have been doubled. Hank and I both had to take time off work, as well as make sure the kids were taken care of. I cannot express how blessed we were to have a place right there in our own community. We truly had the best of the best.

Hank, my late husband, and I both believed that things happen for a reason. The team of doctors assigned to us—that happened for a reason. We believed in them. We believed they wouldn't steer us wrong, and because of this, we got very close to them. They were our friends. We knew they would only recommend to us what they would to their children, wives, or spouses.

March this year marks eight years since Hank passed away. Life has changed a *lot*. I've changed jobs, moved, remarried, started channeling angels . . . So, yeah, a ton of things have changed, but the one thing that has remained the same is that I know I'm right where I'm supposed to be. I felt the same way when I worked for the American Cancer Society. I was in the fight! I was able to get in there, helping and doing everything I could to find a cure, because I don't want anyone to have to go through what I went through. And I don't want my children, or my children's children, to ever hear the words: "You have cancer."

I had friends who lost their husbands around the same time I did. It was interesting to watch each lady react differently. One friend stayed home and never went out much. Another friend took to lots of drinking, while another friend poured her time into her grandson. I realized that I wanted to go out and fight! I was ticked off and working against cancer was a way I could shout it out loud every single day. Working against cancer with the American Cancer Society was healing for me.

Every day I woke up, I knew that Hank was looking down saying, "Go, Honey! You can do it!" Working with the volunteers and everyone who has the passion to beat this darn cancer—believe me, that's what I did. Every day.

I still feel like I get to fight cancer, but now on a different level. With the New You Program, I get to encourage people who are discouraged and help them find their light again. With the help of God and His angels, I still feel like I'm out there fighting against loss and discouragement.

Angel Message From

Archangel Chamuel

Archangel Chamuel is with us right now. After writing the words in Chapter One, Chamuel is coming through very strong—filled with love . . . filled with love. I am very emotional. They are also saying they are all here, but Chamuel is stepping forth to share the teaching of peace—being at peace—also knowing peace comes from remembering that only love is real and that God and angels have so much love for us. No matter what we are going through.

They know that life can be challenging, and that life can throw many wrenches in into the mix. They know that we can sit back and try to understand why . . . why me . . . why this . . . why now . . . why, WHY! The big question of "Why?" as humans comes from a tendency to continue to ask. And Chamuel says, "Why is because you, my dear ones, have asked for this contrast, You have asked for these to be revealed to you, to help you focus on the god within, to help you focus on the love, to help you, dear ones, expand your light, to expand in this lifetime, to expand to a greater level, dear ones. You have asked for this contrast not necessarily in this way or in this manner—it could have been an easier road. It is the road you choose to go down, you can choose this road or you can choose that road. You have chosen this road, dear ones, and the way that you wanted to expand . . . if this makes sense . . . let me elaborate . . .

One does not get disease in the body because they wanted it. We want to clarify this little piece here. It is not because you asked for disease in the body; it is that you wanted to expand at a certain time in your lifetime. Many times, we miss the messages, we miss the mark, we miss the turn, we miss the exit, if you will, we miss the easier road, if you will. We chose to take the road that is the rocky road, the bumpy road, the road less traveled, if you will. We as humans miss the greater exit that would have been the smoother ride.

You, dear Stacie, you went through a lot of rough and tough things as we put it, but you did these things with an angelic presence throughout your life. There were tough times and there were some things that stuck within your physical being that had to be released. As these things are to be released, as these things come to a head, it, as we say, allows for the new road to open up for the detour to be released—the barrier to be moved away, to be moved aside.

For you, dear Stacie, you got right back onto the path and although not understanding all of it, you were back on the path, the path your soul came here to experience. Many people come here to experience things, and they have forgotten we are here as their guardians, as their teams, as Stacie puts it: as their spirit teams who are here to lovingly nudge them, lovingly encourage them, lovingly protect them, and help them. Sending them messages to remind them of where they wanted to be in this lifetime and of their mission. We are always there, we are always a breath away, we are always a prayer away. It is our job to help lovingly guide you. Your spirit team, as Stacie calls it, is never far away. They are always right there, near you, by you, with you.

We are sending you, all of the readers of this book, love from our hearts to yours. We are sending love from the almighty source of God-love that is within all of us. We want you to know we are all connected, we are all tied together, we are all a part of this greater love. We want to remind you that you, too, are going through your journey and you, too, may be experiencing something like disease like Stacie is sharing in her journey.

And we want you to know we are here, you can call upon us, and we will help to guide you back on to the road that is the easier road. We want you to know that this, too, shall pass.

Love to you, dear ones.

Chapter Two

My Diagnosis

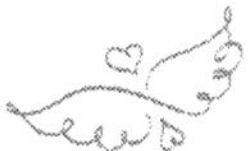

When I was diagnosed with breast cancer, Hank and I had been married for sixteen months. It was February in the year 2005. He was my second husband. I had been married previously to my daughter's father for thirteen years. The relationship was a toxic one and honestly, I should have left two years into it, but I chose not to because I did not believe in divorce. I did love my first husband and, even when I left for brief periods, found myself going back to him until I realized that enough was enough. It was better for both of us that we ended it. This didn't make our divorce easy. With children and thirteen years of baggage between us, the divorce was very messy, but I came through it stronger than I had been before.

I learned from this to do what my heart desired in each moment. Life was too short to hold onto what we would call "limiting beliefs." I needed to follow my gut, my heart, and do what was best for me. As women, we are told we have to please others. I learned to "go for it" and bring my full desires to fruition. Nothing was going to stop me from my happiness. This was the attitude I brought to Hank and our new marriage.

It was Valentine's season and I decided to do something different for Hank. We still considered ourselves newlyweds, and I thought it would be fun to do a boudoir photo shoot. I really wanted to do something special for my wonderful husband, something different, something that was not just a card. On the day of the photo shoot, I went to a friend's studio, and we created some sensual black-and-white shots. Nothing too revealing, but they were sexy and perfect for the bedroom.

For the shoot, I wore a sheer shirt which fully and exquisitely illuminated my left breast—highlighting it in a sensual yet artistic way. Those pictures became quite significant later because at the time of that shoot I had no idea I had cancer. But there I was, showing off my left breast in a sexy photo for my husband. Later we would learn that the photographed breast was the one that had cancer. The pictures were taken before I knew, but I received my diagnosis before the photos were shipped. Seeing those prints was very profound for me because the exposed breast was the one that eventually got removed. Little had I known it was a photo shoot for my breast!

I realized from this that everything happens for a reason in my life. Even this photo shoot was a foreshadowing of what would happen in the future. That picture seemed to signify a date stamp in my life—the point after which everything changed in my life.

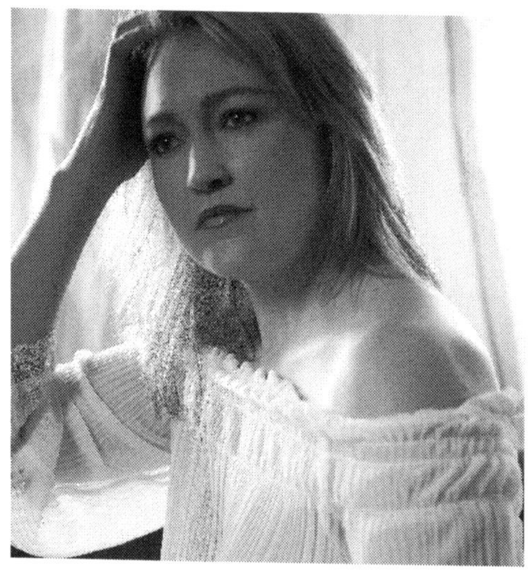

One seemingly normal morning, I walked into work to find my coworkers chatting together in a group. One of the women had just had her mammogram and yearly gynecological appointment, and the girls were making jokes and giggling about it. I'd been putting off my own OBGYN appointment for over two years. It wasn't on purpose, but I was a very busy mom, an account executive, and always moving at full speed. Going in for a checkup, that I didn't really think I needed, never made it to the top of my list.

"Gosh, I need to do that," I added to the conversation.

Just then, Kelly, the one who had been talking about her mammogram, turned to me and asked, "Who's your doctor, Stacie?"

I told her who it was, and Kelly was thrilled. We had the same doctor! Before I knew it, she was dialing the doctor for me. She had the number memorized, so she didn't even have to search for it. Considering how long I'd put off making an appointment, I am almost positive that I never would have called had it not been for Kelly. Knowing how quickly things went from there, I shudder whenever I think about it. God has a way of handling things.

Almost a month passed between that conversation and my appointment. During that period, I had accepted a new job as an ambassador for a company. It was too good to pass up. And it so happened that my very last day of work at my previous job was the day I went and had my checkup. Everything went as usual, and my doctor said, "Let's get a baseline mammogram and get that going for you."

This is also another example of divine intervention. I had made the appointment for that mammogram because I knew my insurance was changing. I literally set it up for the last day that I was employed at my original job. After my mammogram, I returned to the office for my last day, turned in my phone, and gave everything work-related to my old employer. The plan was to go incognito for a week so my new employer could release the news of me coming on board via the media and make a big splash.

However, all does not always go the way you plan. The next day, I had my new phone from my new employer. No one had the number at that point but my family. I was so excited about the new adventure that I headed to the mall for a new business suit. All through that day, my phone kept ringing with wrong-number-type calls. It got so bad that I started ignoring the phone calls until the same number called about six times. At that point, I knew it had to be something important. No one calls six times for nothing. When I finally picked up the phone, it was my doctor.

I was completely shocked that she found my number.

Then she said, "Oh, thank goodness! We got you! This is Doctor . . ."

Meanwhile, I was thinking, Oh my gosh! What's going on? How did she get my number?

She continued, "I've scheduled a mammogram, an ultrasound, and an appointment with the surgeon tomorrow for you."

"Wh-at, wh-at, wh-at, what?!" I stuttered, already panicking.

"Well, we've seen signs of microcalcifications which are signs of carcinoma in your mammogram."

My mind was spinning circles in my head while I grabbed the counter of a mall kiosk. I was breathing so loudly I could hardly hear her words, I was thinking, *What the hell?!* I'd been helping my husband deal with his cancer battle already and now something was wrong with *me*?! I could barely take in the words and held onto the counter feeling disoriented before asking, "Carcinoma?"

"Cancer," she stated.

"Oh... oh, my gosh!" *What was I going to do?* How was I going to battle cancer, help my husband, and have this new job? I was terrified. This was the worst thing that could happen right now, or ever. I had been taking care of everyone else, like most moms, and ignoring myself. Now I would not have a choice.

I frantically found a scrap of paper in my purse so I could write down the information, then hung up and called my husband. I drove to his work to sit with him while we cried together. I did not realize until later that he cried more because he intimately knew the battle I was about to begin. He already had experience with it, and he didn't want me to have to go through that as well.

I did not really know what was about to begin. It is amazing how much struggle a human can go through and survive. I did realize in that moment how much my husband loved and cared for me. When you are going through "hell" you realize who really loves you.

The next day, our journey together began. Both of us battling cancer side by side. How romantic. They diagnosed me with stage two invasive HER2 + breast cancer. I was only 36 years old. They later told me that if I hadn't found it when I did, I wouldn't have made it to my 40th birthday. Sometimes, all of a sudden, you just realize how precious life is and how much you're willing to do to stay alive. You don't take anything for granted anymore.

Until that point, life had felt so good, so simple. I was happily married with three beautiful daughters, and I was in the prime of my career. I was coaching kids' soccer, playing softball, decorating my home, and helping my husband with his cancer journey (which it seemed was getting better; soon he would be getting a six-month break from chemo). It was all happening too fast for me.

Now, my life had turned upside down in a matter of minutes. I was in denial, which is how humans deal with trauma in their lives. I did not feel capable of thinking clearly or handling simple things in my life. It was as if I had shut down mentally and emotionally.

I am truly thankful that I did not have to go to the first surgeon appointment alone. This is because, to this day, I can't remember anything he said. My brain just closed up shop. It is human nature to protect oneself when you mentally can't handle anymore. It is a kind of a defense mechanism. Thankfully, Hank was able to fill me in on the things I was struggling to retain.

Since I was in the middle of a job transition, I was worried I would lose my new opportunity. I immediately went to my former employers and asked if I could still have my old job if my new job did not work out because of my new illness. I was so relieved when they told me that I could! Meanwhile, Hank was at my new employers' office informing them about my situation, and asking if they would still want me working for them. They also said yes! Even though I was very grateful to both my former employers and my new employers, I was still nervous because I wasn't sure if I would be able to give either of them my full one hundred percent.

The first Wednesday in March of that year was my surgery. Then shortly after healing, I was scheduled to start chemotherapy. I talked to the surgeon and asked many questions about what he would be removing. He showed Hank and me the mammogram images on the light board. My left breast looked as though the Milky Way started behind my nipple and went all the way back throughout the milk ducts. It was then I learned that, as pretty as they were, the bright solid white spots were not my friends.

Seeing cancer in your body is a surreal experience. For a second it was like it was happening to someone else. The mammogram was a picture of some other world. I felt apart from it, yet it was affecting so much of my life. I was mystified by how the clusters of small white spots in my breast could have such a large effect on my human experience.

I never felt a lump. I never had symptoms that I would recognize as having breast cancer! The only thing that might have clued me in was the fact I was always exhausted. When it got to about four o'clock each day, I always thought about how wonderful it would feel to crawl under a desk and fall asleep.

We chose to do what the doctor called a skin-sparing quadrant mastectomy. It basically meant they removed the insides of my breast, keeping as much of the skin and nipple as possible—in hopes that reconstructive surgery could simply fill in the missing area, and I would be able to still feel like me. For crying out loud, I was still a newlywed! And to top it all off, we had been trying to have a baby for the last year. I was supposed to be hearing the words, "You are having a baby!" not "You have cancer!"

I kept feeling like I was being robbed. It was like I had done something wrong. I couldn't understand why I was being punished. I was a good person, I always tried to do the right thing, and I was a loving mom, a great wife, and simply loved people. What the hell did I do to deserve this?! I kept having the battle in my mind and in my heart over and over. Every so often, I found myself drifting off with those thoughts, tears rolling down my cheeks. My world as I knew it was no longer mine. I felt like I was living in a foreign body.

I realized hitting what we would call "rock bottom" is what changed my whole life. As much as it hurt, this part of my life was the catalyst for so much change. Without these devastating experiences, I would not be the person I am today. For this, I am forever grateful.

Message from

Archangel Raphael

We are here are today. Archangel Raphael is stepping forth to speak on behalf of the collective of the host of angels.

Ahh, beloved ones, we are here today to give you greetings to encourage you to pay attention to the signs, to pay attention to the thoughts, the ideas that come to you, and the inspiration from loved ones, from friends, from family. We are encouraging you to pay attention to these signs, these are signs of answered prayer, for you—as Stacie has mentioned she would not have booked an appointment for this doctor had it not been for a friend.

We, as your spirit team—as Stacie calls us—as your angels, as your guides, we come to you in many forms. We come to you through friendships, we come to you through families, we come to you through music, we come to you through song, through numbers, through different venues, and we encourage each and every one of you to pay attention to those signs. These are signs that we are trying to get your attention, and we want you to listen, to follow, to trust your intuition.

Trust that knowing—that understanding is within you. Understanding that there are messages—do not distrust those messages, as Stacie puts it, "Do not poo poo those messages."

It is imperative that you learn to trust and you learn to allow these divine messages to come through you. There is a reason that you are receiving these messages and if you are not trusting these messages and going on your merry way, as Archangel Chamuel said earlier, that you will miss that exit, that you will miss that road. It could be a much tougher road.

We are here, constantly sending you messages—divine messages—as our beautiful channel here, Stacie, has a community group about understanding messages. She teaches how to trust and allow. This was one of her most important lessons of learning how to trust and allow, and she has many, many, many experiences in this aspect of learning to trust and allow. Her health was—as she puts it—a redirect of getting her life focused on the mission she is here to accomplish. And we just encourage each and every one of you to pay attention.

As I am also stepping forth to be the host of today's messages coming through the speaker, the coming forth as the presenter, if you will. I also wanted to share that Stacie has had angel activity throughout her entire life and we were never there any more or any less in her journey. It was just that she was allowing and trusting the divine to come through even more. Her faith has always been strong. She has always been a wonderful vessel of God's love, as she puts it.

We have worked through her for many, many, years. For the first time, Stacie was actually really addressing the need for her faith to strengthen and for healing to begin, and we, of course, stepped in and helped her on this divine level. On really looking at herself and what her human body needed. Her soul has always been very connected, but as we are encouraging you, as the readers of this story of the journey that Stacie is sharing with the human collective through her book, you will find us and hear from us along many other avenues throughout your life as well.

We as a collective want you to know that we are here for you, dear ones. We are here . . . We are here . . . You just need to call upon us—call out in prayer, call out asking, knowing that we will be there. Then be allowing, be open, be receptive to receiving, have the belief that you will be healed, have the belief that you are worthy of being healed, dear ones. Beloved, you have a mission and we are here to help you to align with that mission—aligning with the mission allows you to expand in your consciousness, it allows you to expand in this lifetime. This allows us to anchor the light and to help the entire consciousness of the planet. You are all beloved, you are all loved, we are all connected, so being in a state of love-consciousness, we encourage you to go within, to look within, and to remember that it is imperative that you love yourself.

You must love yourself, you must act out self-love. If you are giving love you must receive love. You must be open to loving yourself. We find that the human consciousness, the human side of people have a tendency to, have a—how do we say, forget the necessity of loving oneself? We encourage you, dear ones, to go within and love yourself, to put yourself first, to take care of this human body, to listen to the signs you are receiving, pay attention to the thoughts, pay attention to any ideas that may come to you, because, beloveds, these are answered prayers. These are the answers you have been requesting. These are the answers to questions you may not even know you had. But we encourage you, beloveds, to trust, to allow, and to go within and have self-love. To begin that healing—that sacred journey of healing—so that you may expand, so that you may experience that which you, dear ones, wanted to experience in this lifetime. We are here to help you stay aligned with your mission.

And so it is.

Chapter Three

Friend-Date

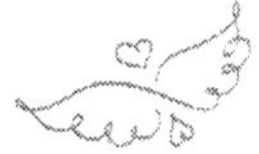

In 2003, before Hank and I got married, we were friends.

Hank had been my softball coach from 1992 to 1998, when I joined his team, the Plate Smashers. I found out he had cancer and that he had been given only six months to live. Mutual friends also told me he was likely to die in his upcoming debulking surgery. And so, I helped arrange a fundraiser to help his family, which eventually raised $3,500.

One day, I picked him up for lunch because I had the freedom to drive all over town with my job. We went to Olive Garden, then I drove him back to his office in Eugene, Oregon. He was only in his thirties, but he was walking like he was ninety. The sight broke my heart. As he got out of the car he leaned his head back into it, looked into my eyes, and said: "Batter up."

His words made me break into uncontrollable sobs because it was an inside joke from our softball days. We'd first become friends when I played had played co-ed softball against his team for a few years. Both of our teams were ranked top, always neck and neck. One year, he decided he was going to make an undefeated team. And that was how he got me to join his team. As the coach, he would say, 'Batter up,' and though everything was stacked against us, we would still win. I had heard him say these words many times before, but this time, it was heart-wrenching. It was as if he was preparing to move on to the next thing if he had to. His next big game.

I didn't see him for a while after that. Time passed, my divorce was finalized, and I didn't even know how he was doing. And then, suddenly, he called. Unfortunately, he called my old line, the one in the house my ex still lived in. Back then, my ex was really irritated. In a grumpy voice, my ex called and told me that some guy was calling for me. It was after our divorce and his exact words were, "Your *coach* called. You better get him your new number!"

And that was it. I didn't even mind the bitterness of his words. I was so glad to hear that Hank was still alive. I had been utterly out of touch with him during the divorce and had no idea how he was doing. I called him immediately and we got to talking. I was so happy he was doing well. I told him about my divorce, and he told me that when he went into his debulking surgery, he wasn't supposed to survive. His wife had not visited; instead, she had divorce papers delivered to him. The phone call led to us both talking about our children, and we realized without the kids' constant schedule, we had some matching days to go on a friend-date together.

We met at a sports bar and started talking about how we were going to get back into the dating world, something neither of us had been involved in for years. And then, he asked the mind-blowing question: "Well, you wouldn't go on a date with me, would you?"

Truly, my mind was blown. I couldn't believe I had not even considered it. That was the beginning of everything.

Hank had a rare form of gastrointestinal cancer. He'd actually been diagnosed at the same time we'd been on a softball team together. He told me later that he'd swung the bat one day and felt something in his stomach "tear like Velcro." It might have felt like a tear, but what was really happening was that a thick mass of cancer was growing inside him, and now it was beginning to interfere with normal movement. The cancer mass had likely started in his appendix, but by the time they found it, there was so much, and it was so widespread that they couldn't say exactly where it had started.

When the doctors finally diagnosed Hank's cancer, they gave him six months to live—but that was if he did nothing. The debulking surgery was one of the options they gave him as an alternative to sitting around waiting to die. The goal was to try to take a lot of the bulk of that cancer out and then start treatments with chemotherapy. That was the road that he chose to take. Mind you, before he got to that point, four doctors turned him away. They said, "No, there's nothing we can do for you," or "It's too late," and "You're in stage four."

Looking back, I realize life was preparing me for my future with cancer. The relationship I had with Hank supported me through one of the hardest times of my life. Without him, I do not think I would have survived. I am forever grateful for Hank and the lessons he taught me in this incarnation.

It was amazing how he found the doctor who took the step. He was explaining his situation to a woman who worked for the surgeon, and he physically drew a picture of what his cancer looked like on a napkin. She took it back to the office and shared it with the surgeon who then told her that he wanted to see Hank. Hank went to see him, and together, they decided to go ahead and try.

Divine intervention? I believe so. The universe brought Hank a miracle and was able to guide him to the healing he desired. I believe that when we have a strong desire for something, the universe will aid us in so many ways. It's magical how this universe works.

The surgeons went in and did a debulking surgery. They removed five pounds of cancerous tissue. It was like a weight belt—it was twenty-some inches long, five inches wide, and about a half an inch thick. It was all wrapped around in his omentum—in the stomach area like mesh netting that kind of held everything together. It was a great success. This surgery alone extended his life tremendously.

He started chemotherapy, just to hammer it down, and he did really well. After his first chemo session, he lost a lot of weight. He was very, very skinny. He walked around like he was about thirty years older than he was. But he was happy to be alive. Hank's children, when he was diagnosed, were ages two and three, so his goal was to be a great father and to be there long enough for them to remember him. So he was going to do anything he had to do to make that happen.

In fact, Dr. Monticelli even said, "Hank's case, I think, was a little bit unique. In part, because of his determination and his health. He was able to sustain so much more treatment than a lot of other patients do."

Hanks's strong desire to live is what kept him alive. He had such strong willpower which resulted in him feeling alive and well. He desired so much for his children to remember him that he was able to overcome impossible odds. When we are committed and desire something with our full being, we can move mountains.

He fought cancer for about a year before we started dating. At that point, he was on a six-month break from chemo. In those six months, he was doing really great—playing softball and just living life. We both loved softball so much that for our first date we decided to go out for a bite to eat after playing together. But by the time our game ended, everything was closed, so I invited him back to my house. We took our cleats off and sat there talking. I walked him to the front door of my home to see him out, and he leaned down to kiss me. Just as he did, a little thought that sprung to my mind was, *I hope this won't make softball awkward.*

I was panicking! Here was this handsome man, who I would soon learn was my soulmate, leaning in to kiss me and I was too busy worrying about our recreational social life! Hank assured me that nothing would be awkward, and when he kissed me, I knew it was true. During this first kiss, I knew I wanted to be with him. Something in my heart expressed, "This is the man for you." I always trust my intuition when it comes to making a decision, and I am glad I trusted it that time.

I want to explain more about trusting your intuition in the moment. During the span of our lives, our angels are providing us with guidance. When we trust the impulses our angels provide us, our lives flow with more ease. Trusting our impulses leads to miracles, such as my relationship with Hank.

By August, four weeks later, we were officially dating. He was working for an advertising agency and we headed to Salem, Oregon. He was filming a commercial for McGrath's Fish House and I was in it. We said "I love you" for the first time at the hotel. You see, I had already been thinking about how much I wanted to tell him I loved him, and I was trying to pony up the courage to just do it. I decided to go for it while we were about to fall asleep in the hotel room, but he beat me to it. He said he had something to tell me, and I said, "I do, too." We were both about to say: 'I love you." How perfect is that?

Looking back, I really think we were twin flames. Even though I had known him for about eleven years already, there was something about him that summer that I couldn't put my finger on. When I looked at him it made my heart flutter. I wanted to cry because I was so thankful he was still alive. He had always been my friend and my softball coach. Now he had become something more, the man I loved. It was like he had gone to war and came back a hero.

A twin flame is someone who comes into our lives to help us grow exponentially in our lifetimes. Our twin flame usually appears during an important moment—such as when we are diagnosed with cancer. They are usually in our lives for a short period of time to catalyze rapid growth. Hank was this for me. I would not be where I am currently without him. I hope he gets to read this.

Dr. Monticelli also mentioned, "But a lot of it also is the expectations and the determination of a patient. Some people would quit based on the side effects a lot sooner than he did."

Every time a new drug came out, Hank's doctor, Dr. Monticelli, would contact us. He had connections all over the country giving him details on what the new drugs were and how they could help. He was researching and finding drugs that would help Hank because it was a rare form of cancer, and they didn't know a lot about it. He would inform us of his new discoveries and keep us in the loop so we could find the best path for Hanks's healing. We got to do our research on each drug and make an informed decision as to what we were going to do.

According to Dr. Monticelli, "We were able to push a little bit harder, a little bit longer, bring in some newer agents. Part of that was his physiology. Part of that, I like to think, was that I was able to mix and match drugs in a fashion that allowed us to get things in that were active but not too toxic. He really went through as much therapy as I've given somebody in the past decade."

That was the nice thing about the Willamette Valley Cancer Center. They were always open, the doctor was always willing to try a new idea. If we heard about something that worked, they would always check it out, and then we would make an informed decision together. I always felt like the staff was our team of champions in this battle.

I believe Hank's determination to get better attracted the best doctors to him. They were willing to go the distance because he was. I am forever grateful for the Willamette Valley Cancer Center. I believe my angels guided us there.

Hank asked me to marry him during our first softball game in September. Everything seemed normal, and it was a regular game. I was up to bat, getting ready for the pitch, and the ump yelled, "BATTER'S OUT! Batter is out for wearing jewelry!"

I looked at him, shock written on my face. I did not have to look to know that I was not wearing jewelry. But he yelled it over and over which annoyed me further. I was particularly angry because I was tired of dealing with so many aggressive men at that time in my life. I argued with him, but it was no use.

The ump only yelled in response, "Take it up with the coach!"

So, I looked to Hank for help, but instead of coming to my aide, he slowly meandered out into the field, taking his sweet time. Frustrated beyond belief, I turned back to the umpire to continue arguing my case and, while I was doing that, I saw Hank was on one knee! My mouth fell open—but it wasn't because I finally understood what was happening; I was shocked and appalled that he was goofing around instead of helping me! Annoyed, I motioned to the umpire and turned back to Hank saying, "What are you doing? Quit messing around! Get off the ground and take care of this!" But then, I saw the ring and I went from fury to total love as he asked me to marry him over home plate.

He pulled a brand new batter's glove out of his back pocket. "You need a glove to put over the ring because jewelry is not allowed," Hank told me, and I just grinned like an idiot.

He had obviously planned it all with the ump. I could hear rustling and murmuring all around me as spectators were trying to figure out if I was really out or not.

"Is she really out?"

"What's going to happen now?"

This continued until the ump finally shouted, "Okay, batter up."

Then came the best part; I hit the ball over the fence and got a home run! What a perfect finale for that spectacular event in my life.

When we went home for the night, he said to me, "I'm sorry if that was too kooky for you."

"Oh no, go ahead and keep it up because I just fell deeper in love with you," I told him. And I meant it. Too kooky? No way! I was so in love with him!

This was one of the best moments of my life. Hank was so sweet and knew me so well. I look back at that experience in my mind all the time. The fact I hit a home run afterward makes it all the more special. These moments of light in the darkness are what keep us going as humans. If we can focus on these during our dark times, we can get through anything.

Because the cancer was growing very fast, and he resumed chemo, we decided to get married quickly. In our own nervousness, we invited the pastor and his wife over for dinner Sunday night to share with them all the reasons we felt we shouldn't get married yet and all the reasons we also felt we needed to get married right away. We needed to weigh the pros and cons. By the end of the evening, we were all convinced we needed to be married right away. We knew that God's plans for us were great. We got married a week later, the weekend after Thanksgiving. It was a humble little affair, but to our surprise, the church was completely packed, even with such short notice.

Message from

Archangel Gabriel

We are here, and Archangel Gabriel is stepping up to speak on behalf of the host of angels today.

Ah, dear ones, dear ones, we encourage each and every one of you to take the time to nurture that inner child in you. As Stacie shares on her journey, the love of playing softball together is a time of being playful, a time of being silly, a time of being able to be childlike. And with the beautiful story of her journey and her beloved one, Hank, of how he proposed marriage during a time of childlike play.

Of course, there was love. Of course, there was more love that expanded the love between both of them, and as her journey shares that she believes they were twin flames.

Twin Flames are all about finding and reconnecting on this earth plane. They are all about helping each other to heal the wounded heart. To heal, to be able to expand and transform into a more expanded awakened being—so that is, as we say, beautiful. Beautiful, dear ones, beautiful work upon this earth, beautiful in helping each other expand and heal.

And we say that miracles do happen; miracles happen every day, countless times a day, every second, every minute, every hour, miracles are happening. Believe and you shall receive, dear ones. Believe and you shall receive. It is happening all around you—the gifts that are awaiting your opening, dear ones.

Do not withhold from the love that is coming to you. Allow yourself to open and receive these gifts, dear ones. Open your arms and receive. If it takes time for you to be childlike, live childlike, create time and space for you to be playful, be silly, laugh, and enjoy doing things that you are not so stressed and worried about. The particulars—every day—day in and day out—it is imperative to nurture the inner child.

Allow that inner child to come out and play. Allow the time needed to heal your heart, heal the wounds that have happened, heal so that the walls may melt away and that you can expand that love and give a greater sense to the entire world.

And so it is—we say—blessed, beloved ones.

Chapter Four

Put on a Happy Face

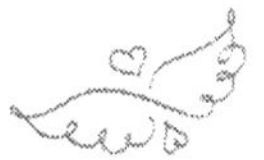

My beautiful daughter, Alex, said tearfully a few years ago, "I'm 17. I'll be 18 in September. Hank and Stacie are my mom and my step-dad. When my mom got it, when she was diagnosed, that's when I kinda understood, okay, this is really serious."

They wanted to perform a biopsy to make sure they knew exactly what they needed to remove and from where. That was my first step to getting the crap out of my body. I was scared to death. I was informed, after putting my gown on, that Hank could not go with me. For the first time, I felt truly alone. I had always had a tendency to live by the 'fake it till I make it' rule or to put on that happy face even though, inside, I was dying. However, that day, I found that those ways of coping were all fine and dandy for your career, but now shit was real and it was not working for me!

In our society, we are forced to put on a "happy face" and ignore our emotions. This leads to disease in our bodies as the emotional debris has been building up over time. When we are willing to face our emotions the true healing can begin, which happened in my surgery. Angels are telling us it is okay to feel whatever we are feeling. We are loved by God no matter how angry, sad, or fearful we are. We are always blessed by Source.

I entered a tiny doctor's office that had a table for me to lie down on. There was this one big hole in the table—odd. I had never seen a table like that before. They started an IV and gave me something to make me loopy, which hit right away. Thank God! There were about four people in the room with me and they all sat on the rolling stools close to the floor. They asked me to place my left breast into the hole in the table, then they raised the table up, and all slid underneath me.

This was so weird! My mind was racing nine hundred miles a minute, and I kept thinking of how it was like getting your oil changed in the car. I couldn't see what they were doing and I was disoriented and not feeling much at that point, but I just remember hearing the sounds of a machine that reminded me of a sewing machine, along with a tugging sensation of my breast. This was the machine removing samples for them to test.

Crank the table up, roll the doctors under so they could work on my undercarriage, right? Crank the table back down and give her a test drive! A few times, they had me get up and stand at the mammogram machine so they could find the next area that needed to be removed. I had a drinking-straw-size hole right above my areola on top of my breast. You know how, on tropical islands, they poke a hole in a coconut and stick in a straw before they hand it to you? That's what my breast looked like! Once they felt they got what they needed, they put a stitch in me, and I was headed back home.

Even though I can laugh and make light of that experience now, I was terrified when I was on that table. It hit me that this was real, and this surgery would be the make-or-break for me. I prayed and asked for guidance to allow my healing to unfold with ease and grace. I felt my angels by my side giving me encouragement. I was so supported by the four people in the room and Source bringing support from all angles. Looking back, I was at the divine perfect place, but that did not keep me from being scared out of my mind!

It was the first Wednesday in March that I had the first surgery. To my shock, it was more like a drive-through mastectomy. I checked in that morning at Sacred Heart Medical and was sent home by one o'clock that afternoon.

My daughter, Alex, reflected back and said, "I felt like I was going to lose my mom. I didn't really know what to do. I had never had to deal with that. I had never had anyone in my family that had to deal with it, so it was kind of shocking."

We chose to do a quadrant mastectomy. That meant we were basically saving part of the breast and removing everything behind and underneath, with the understanding that if that could not happen, we would remove the entire breast.

"She took her diagnosis quite well. I think some of that may have had to do with the fact that she already knew a lot about cancer and the treatments. Hank, at that time, was probably a great source of support for her because he knew exactly what she was dealing with." This was what Dr. Monticelli said sometime later.

During my first surgery, they removed a portion of cancer. It was not a lump; it was not anything I could feel, but it was there. When I looked at the mammogram sheets up on the lighted board, I could see that it followed the duct from one end all the way to the back. During the mastectomy, they scooped that out and did something like a lumpectomy. They hoped they had it all.

As I was in the recovery room from surgery, something strange happened. I had not yet "come to," but I recall hearing multiple voices calling my name over and over. They sounded a million miles away! That didn't bother me because I remember feeling so much peace and love and being so content where I was. But the more I heard my name, the more I was alerted to my surroundings. It felt like I was drifting in a long, somewhat dark tunnel. To say it was black doesn't really describe it. I could see, so it was not like a black dark night. But there were walls that made it appear like a spherical tunnel with a dark space in it. I saw a light ahead but it seemed a very long way away.

A smooth motionless, weightless feeling gradually pulled me toward a warm glow I could see ahead. I felt no stress, no worries, no thoughts whatsoever. I just was and I felt wonderful. For some reason, hearing my name called didn't pique my interest too much. It really felt like it was too far away to even bother with acknowledging it. Then all of sudden, I felt a falling sensation, or like I was being sucked backward. The feeling only seemed like a split second! I found myself gasping for air, my heart pounding out of my chest as if I had just run a race. People were around me, but I was too confused to process anything.

A doctor was holding my hand and patting it over and over while calling my name, "Stacie, wake up, Stacie, wake up!" A couple of nurses also called my name. I sensed there were several faces huddled over me. The first thing I recall actually seeing was the large cross outside the window on the other side of the hospital. I remember thinking to myself, *Am I in heaven?*

The sunlight was shining on the cross so beautifully I wondered if that was the light I had just been moving toward.

To this day, I am not completely sure what happened on the "outside"—in the recovery room when they almost lost me. I know that I coded—for a few moments I lost my heartbeat and the doctors and nurses had to administer a medication to bring me back. I do not know what was put in my IV to get my heart to do what it did, but it brought me back from my drifting away from my body. Nothing like this ever happened again in my other my surgeries.

After this experience, my life was changed. I felt closer to the life beyond. And I felt closer to the angels all around us. I began to hear and feel them speaking to me. It was my first experience with heavenly angels.

Angelic comfort or not, I still had cancer and it needed to be dealt with. About three days after that first surgery, the results came back. They weren't as we hoped. Instead of completely removing the cancer, they'd merely cut through it. And so the next Wednesday, I went back in for another surgery. They went back in through the same incision. They thought they'd gotten it all this time. They thought we were all good. But three days later, the results came back again. This time, they revealed that there was cancer in the first lymph node, so once again, we scheduled another surgery for the following Wednesday. It was clear at this point that I had Stage Three cancer, which brought more worry to me and my family. Every Wednesday in the month of March in 2005, I was in surgery.

Alex said, "My mom had one surgery after another for a couple of weeks. It was hard. It was weird. I'd never had surgery; I'd never broken a bone. I'd never really had to go through that. And I'd never really seen Hank go through surgery because he did his surgery before my mom got married to him. So it was kinda weird - new for me."

I can't even imagine how scary and hard it must have been for my daughter! Being 15, she was dealing with some very grown-up stuff—stuff I wish I could have protected her from. I knew I had to be strong for her and I had to beat this cancer! I could not stand the thought of not being there for her. I am so proud of her; she was everything to me!

I felt so much guilt for allowing my daughter to support me. My mind kept on saying "Why did I put my daughter through this?!" However, I knew in my heart this was meant to be, and she was strong and willing to support me through this difficult time. It is interesting how our heart knows one thing but our mind says another. This is why it is so important to connect with our hearts on a daily basis.

I feel that the last surgery was the toughest mentally and emotionally. My mom traveled again to be with me. And that time, my dad came in, too, from Nevada. It was in those times I felt like saying some profound thing. But just being in the presence of my family seemed to be enough. I know it had to be hard for each of them to watch. Being their child, I can only imagine what they were feeling.

I was so supported through this process. I believe God gives us exactly what we need when we need it. Source is always there for us in our time of need. Thank God my family was there for me. Inside I was a mess, but I continued to stay strong for them as much as I could. I am forever grateful for the support they gave me that day.

The hardest part was the prep work going into the operating room. I was inside a mammogram machine for what seemed like about an hour. They gave me a chair to sit on and lowered down the machine, but there was really nowhere to put my arms. It was *so* uncomfortable! My back cramped up, and I had to keep taking shallow breaths.

Quiet tears streamed down my face, all the while my breast was smashed inside the grips of this cold and uncaring machine I was hugging. They were trying to find exactly where the margins of the cancer were. When they found the spot behind the nipple, they injected a numbing agent and then put a needle inside to mark that area. They then did the same thing near the back part closest to my chest wall. After this was done, they put paper-drinking cups over the needles so no one would get poked. I looked like a medical Madonna-wannabe.

As the time went by, the medication started to wear off and I began to feel. It was getting more and more painful by the moment. Burning, sharp, shooting pains ran through my breast. It got so bad I had tears flowing down my face by the time they were able to get me more pain meds. Soon after that, I was wheeled into surgery.

Hank was a TV producer. He documented darn near everything—good and bad. He wanted his daughters to be able to have the memories if he ever had to leave this world. When I went in for this final surgery, the camera was rolling once again. I am so thankful for him capturing so much on video so that I can share my story. It has also helped me to recall the details more clearly.

With surgery, they went in, actually removing the lining off my pec muscle—just like you would remove the lining from the back of a rack of ribs. They also went in and removed nineteen more lymph nodes underneath my arm. Before they did this, they added some kind of radioactive material into my lymph nodes so they could find it later with the Geiger counter. It all seems so *Incredible Hulk* sometimes—like I was moving from one experiment to another.

They knew by then that because they would be removing so many of my lymph nodes, I was going to need a portacath installed. This gives IV access under the skin to draw blood and give treatments. The reason I needed it was that—due to the surgeries—the veins of one of my arms would be too weak to withstand the chemo drugs. They placed the device about three fingers below my collarbone and directly above my right breast. It was almost a quarter-size circle directly under my skin, like a large button with a flat surface. Running from that was a long tube that connected up to my heart. That was where the chemo was to be administered instead of through my arms.

When I woke up after that last surgery, something was different. I was not in the large general ward with bed after bed, and no one was forcing me to go to the bathroom and swap out my bed for a chair. The hustle and bustle were absent. In fact, I was surrounded by all my family and had my own hospital room. Everything was fuzzy. and I was not sure what happened. I did try to get up and use the restroom. On my way there, I found that I could hardly breathe. It seemed like a miracle that I made it back to the bed. I felt like there was an elephant sitting on my chest. Soon after that, the doctor came in to tell us what happened.

He said, "Remember how I mentioned there was a slim chance that your lung could get punctured when they placed the portacath into your chest? Well, unfortunately, that is what happened."

What!?

According to the doctor, I had to stay overnight or even longer, until my lung fixed itself. (Yes, apparently lungs fix themselves!) Throughout the night, every two hours they took me to X-ray to make sure it was healing. I could see the fear in my daughters' eyes. Their precious little hearts were wondering if Mommy was going to make it back home.

"Seeing her on the hospital bed, all groggy, and ya know how that is. It was really different. It was kinda hard, but I don't think, at the time, I really knew what to expect or think or feel. It was just, as long as she was able to get in and get out alive and healthier or with less cancer than when she went in, the better," said Alex.

When I finally got to go home, I could not walk well by myself. I had to have help to tackle the stairs to our bedroom. I remember getting to the third or fourth step and having to stop and wait like I was eighty years old! It was that day, after living in that home for over a year, I realized, *Damn, I have nineteen steps to get to my bed!* I never counted the steps before or even thought about them much. But at that moment, as I faced my nineteen stairs, I realized how limited I was. I might not be able to make it to the kitchen, see my daughters off to school, or carry a basket of laundry. I went from being Superwoman to needing help in more ways than I ever imagined. Up to that point, that month was truly the hardest thing I had ever endured. I couldn't imagine it getting worse. I knew then and at that moment that I could not do it by myself!

As a mom, it is so hard to accept help from others. We are so used to taking care of others in our day-to-day lives. I felt helpless during this time and worthless to my daughters. For all the moms out there: show your emotions and let yourself be human. I believe we hold so much to be the "perfect mom" in the world. However, we do not have to feel guilty for going through this human experience, feeling emotions, and being weak sometimes. We are allowed the same obstacles and struggles as anyone else.

Message from

Archangel Raziel

Archangel Raziel is stepping forth to speak on the behalf of the collective today.

There have been many signs and many more will be given whenever anyone is going through these trials in this human incarnation. Many times, when we experience a thinning of the veil there will be an increased awareness that will shift your relationships, will shift your goals in life, will shift and redirect—as Stacie puts it—on to your soul's mission.

Helping to mirror what your life should look like to reflect what your soul is going through and what your soul is needing to go through to fulfill in this lifetime. Dear ones, we want you to know you are never alone, even though life can feel very lonely, especially when going through tough, tough times.

Dear ones, we know that it is hard to experience something such as Stacie has gone through with her surgeries and her physical body manifesting disease. But we encourage you to know you have never been alone, you are always . . . always in the presence of God and our team of angels. We are always there for you, dear ones. You have never been alone—this entire life you have never been alone. We are right there with you, for you, and around you at all times.

We will, dear ones, use this experience to help you to realign with your soul's mission. This is very important that you start to remember, and that you see the signs. Pay attention to the signs. We will be helping you by sending and providing more information. This is a way that we began working with Stacie more . . . this disease that she went through. The experience slowed her life down. Slowed her down where she focused on what is truly important.

Our advice to you, dear ones, is to learn how to be. How to be, how to listen, how to just be in the moment so you do not get yourself into a place of having to deal with the disease in your human, physical body. When you can be in a place of being, in the stillness, you will receive, you will hear, you will know, and you will be guided in a much easier way to getting on track with your soul's mission.

We, as a collective, are sending love to you, dear ones.

Sending much-needed love.

Much needed love to you.

And so it is.

Chapter Five

Trading Places

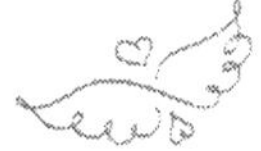

For the first time, I found myself going to Willamette Valley Cancer Center as a patient rather than just as Hank's caregiver. I had been going there for a year and a half with my husband every other week. I knew the nurses, the staff at the front desk, the doctor. I had been the caregiver, doing everything I was supposed to do—and now I suddenly had to have treatment myself!?

I was used to taking care of others so it was odd to care of myself. I have learned over time, as a mother and woman, I need to learn how to receive. We cannot give love unless we are willing to receive love in return. This would be like God not receiving our love and worship. As mothers, we are required to receive from others to be at our full self. I was finally able to receive when I was going through cancer treatment.

Dr. Monticelli said I had a relatively aggressive form of cancer, so they had to treat it with an aggressive form of chemotherapy. After a year and a half of being there, the hospital staff members were like my extended family, so when they learned I would now be a patient, I got many hugs. A couple of nurses had tears in their eyes. They were sad that I had to go through treatments. But I knew that was the place I needed to be. They were my family—they were in the battle with me. I felt so supported when I was there. It was as if divine guidance put me in the perfect place at the perfect time.

I almost felt like the folks at the cancer center had this newfound fight in them because it was not fair that a husband and wife were going through this at the same time. I believe our determination, together, helped us to get through it. I noticed our energy was rubbing off on them, which gave them a fighting spirit.

> *Even Dr. Monticelli said, "So this was definitely the first time I've treated a husband and a wife at the same time. I've treated family members before, but again, never simultaneously."*

I just sort of felt like they scooped us up in their arms and held us when we couldn't walk on our own. I felt so supported by these amazing individuals. Each day, their smiles uplifted my spirit and kept me going. In a way, this hospital became my community and tribe, which helped me get through one of the hardest times of my life.

Dr. Monticelli was my husband's oncologist, and when it was time for my surgeon to recommend an oncologist to us, my husband said, "No, no. She's going to see, Dr. Monticelli."

Dr. Monticelli even said it was pretty clear our roles were going to be reversed for that time period. In the patient room, I was sitting on the table, and my husband was sitting on the chair for the first time. It was very surreal, or maybe it was more like being hit by a truck. Sometimes I even thought, *You've got to be kidding me! This has to be a joke.* I could hardly believe this happened to both of us. But Dr. Monticelli was very positive. It was also at that moment that I thought about how on earth anyone could go through this without faith. I do not believe I could have done it without being able to rely on God's strength to get me through.

I believe, in each moment we are guided by our angels. In these moments, I relied on my spiritual strength. Without my faith in God, I would not have been able to survive. When we rely on the angels surrounding us we can get through anything. My faith in God is my greatest weapon, and I used it constantly during my struggle with cancer.

Dr. Monticelli did a good job of not giving us false hope or unrealistic expectations. A big part of what he does is helping a patient find those realistic expectations. In fact, he tells it like it is—here are the statistics, here's what has happened, here's what could happen, here's what might happen. He laid it all out and answered questions over and over. For me personally, because I was so overwhelmed, I think I only retained maybe 10 percent, so thank goodness Hank was able to have a level head and listen! He told me things later that Dr. Monticelli said because, to be honest, several times, I was like, "I don't remember that! What? Where was I?" But overload was to be expected. The reality was still sinking in. For me, I just kind of checked out. But I've been told that was normal. The blinds would close, and I would become starry-eyed and gaze into space.

That made me realize just how important a caregiver is. To have or be that support person is priceless. Hank told me he had to go to some of his appointments alone before we got together. He would take a tape recorder and record everything the doctor said so he could play it back whenever he needed.

Those recordings also become helpful to me at times, too.

When you are going through a struggle it is so important to have another person to lean on. When we have to do things alone, we lose faith, which, in turn, allows us to fail. I think when we have another person who can stay level-headed, they can help us to see the light and keep up our strength. I recommend anyone going through hardship to find someone to lean on, even if you have to seek outside help.

Knowing that our roles were about to be reversed made me worry about how the kids would be taken care of, how the meals would be cooked, and the house cleaned. I worried about Hank's cancer coming back and his treatments needing to be much stronger again. What would happen if neither of us could do all those things? I worried about missing work and having less income. I worried about losing our insurance if we didn't keep working. I stressed a lot over not being able to do the job my employer expected. Deep down, I truly thought my job was more important than taking care of me. Simply put, I worried a whole lot.

Of course, I know now that worrying so much only made everything worse. But, if we tune in and acknowledge our worry, instead of giving in to it, it helps us to connect deeper to God and our inner selves. I believe I got closer to God through my experience with cancer. This is much easier to say when looking back, however, in the moment I was scared and terrified. Through this crazy process with my twin flame, I was able to find my true self, and now I am living out my purpose in an amazing and heart-centered way. I am thankful I am able to help people due to the struggles I went through.

Message from

Archangel Zadkiel

We are here, dear ones. Archangel Zadkiel is stepping forth feeling lots of love... lots of love... a warm, glowing, heartfelt beam of love coming from the collective, the host of angels.

Not only do the angels have a ton of compassion for all of us who are going through these tough times, they are also encouraging us to have compassion for ourselves, for others, but mostly for ourselves. Really coming at it from a loving heart is going to empower us for change, empower us to get through these tough times.

Archangel Zadkiel is helping us and anyone who is going through such deep emotional struggles due to disease or any kind of health concern or any emotional issues for that matter. Helping us to heal on an emotional level so we can bring miracles into play. Deep...

deep emotional healing is what the angels are asking us to focus on so we can get through to the next level.

Encouraging us to really use the power we have within us, setting the intention to be able to manifest a healthy body, to be able to manifest all the blessings that we deserve in this life. Be really able to muster up all the strength within us and take back our power so we can have the authority to manifest healing—as God wants us to have this healing.

We need to stand in our power and receive these blessings... receive... reminding us to give away the fear. Allow the angels and our spirit teams to take that, reverse those feelings, and know that God has our backs, and know God is taking care of us. God has assigned us these beautiful angels—beautiful spirit teams—to lift us up, hold us underneath each arm, and help us to walk when we feel we cannot walk.

Release this pain, dear ones, and go within to heal on an emotional level so that you can manifest the new you, the new reality, and see yourself as healed. BELIEVE that your SELF is healed. KNOW that your SELF is healed. Open your arms to receive God's gifts for you, await the reveal, untie the bow, open the lid, remove the tissue, and pull out the gift. RELISH in the gift. RECEIVE the gift, dear ones. RECEIVE the gift. You are worthy of this gift. God has this gift waiting just for you. Set your intentions and manifest great health and manifest great healing and RECEIVE the gift.

And so it is.

Chapter Six

Chemo-Dates

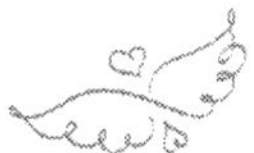

My doctors decided chemo was the best action to take first because we were going to try to shrink anything that was left in there after the surgeries. We were going to hit it hard because I was young.

"Then once we do chemo, we are going to switch over and do radiation, just as a precaution. Let's just make sure that it's gone," Dr. Monticelli told me. He also told me chemotherapy was medicine designed to kill the growing and dividing cells. That is exactly what a cancer is: a disturbance of cellular growth. Chemotherapy targets those processes by preventing cell growth which is how it stops cancer cells.

The scary thing was wondering what was going to happen—the unknown. How bad was it going to be? Was it going to hurt? What would it feel like?

Because you just don't know. Everyone is different. Really, my only knowledge about the whole process came from watching Hank go through his treatment. My understanding was that it was bad! However, every drug combination gives folks different side effects as well. I had heard of a lady doing a form of chemo that was simply a pill she took daily. It caused her to have IBS (Irritable Bowel Syndrome) and a little tiredness, but for the most part, she was totally fine. For her, it was basically life as normal.

I have learned it is important to dive into the unknown and trust my angels and spirit guides. The best way to dive into the unknown is to allow life to work out for you. You do this by following your intuition in each moment. When I am working with my angel guides, I am connecting with my heart chakra, which is the emotional center. By connecting with our emotional centers, we are able to follow our inner guidance, which shows us the best possible action to take. So if your heart tells you to trust the chemo, do it.

For my first round of chemo, Hank was well enough that he didn't have to do it with me, thank goodness. I sat in his favorite chair and it was very scary. I was very glad I knew everyone on staff and everyone knew who we were. I knew the routine already, so I knew I could get a juice box, and I knew

I could sit in my chair, and I knew I could watch a movie with a cuddly blanket.

Dr. Monticelli prescribed me a cocktail of drugs that he said could really knock somebody down for several months. It was called the dose-dense chemotherapy or DDC for short. It is a combination of drugs administered in a specific order and style that aims to achieve maximum tumor kill ratio for those of us with HER2 positive tumors and positive lymph nodes (estrogen driven). I would also be starting a drug called Herceptin. Mind you, I am not a doctor nor have I studied as a doctor. I am simply sharing with you my knowledge and understanding of these drugs and how they worked, based on my experience.

Dr. Monticelli told me chemotherapy, in general, could make a person feel anywhere from somewhat tired to extremely run down. Nausea was usually not a big problem, but it could be, depending on the age of the patient and what kind of chemo they were getting. For me, it was. It caused me to be in horrible pain and sick all the time. I would never wish that kind of pain on anyone. But Hank and I had a motto we lived by: "*What you think about you bring about.*" So we tried very hard to always think positive. A lot of the cancer fight is how you perceive it in your mind. You just have to think positive. It will help you kick cancer's butt! If you give up mentally, cancer for sure will take over. So I set positive affirmations. Cancer was NOT stopping me!

I hold my kids in my arms . . .

I play softball every week . . .

I work full time at my job . . .

I am healthy and happy . . .

The key to overcoming anything in life is to have a positive mindset. I have been told by my angels to keep a positive mindset over and over again. Our thoughts have the ability to change our whole lives for the better or worse. If I did not have this positive mindset I would never have been able to beat cancer.

My friend Cheri mentioned, "She's one of the strongest people that I have ever been around. Going through the kind of treatment she was going through – you could tell it was taking a toll on her but she was never going to admit that."

One of our RNs, Susan said, "It was a tough time in the chemo room for the two of them. I think it's a bonding time but I think it's also a really rough time because they have a family to go home to that they had to care for."

Eventually, Hank needed another round of chemo as well. When this happened, we planned our treatments together, every other Friday. We held hands and sat in the chairs together and watched a movie. At times, we joked that we were headed to date night together. Too bad we were not able to get a mani-pedi at the same time. Heck, we were already getting our fill of a specialty mixed cocktail.

The laughter and joy we brought to our sessions were really healing for us and the staff around us. At times, I think our humor was the greatest gift we gave each other. Without those laughs, we would never have made it through chemotherapy, and I think we would have given up.

Dr. M. said in an interview for the WVCI blog, "The thing I remember the most about them is they were both such upbeat people that the staff and other patients looked forward to having them there."

As much as I hated going to my chemo appointments, I always loved the people. Seeing other patients there not only helped me to remember, *if they can do it, so can I*, but also, I realized later on that we were just as much of an inspiration to each of them.

There was one particular gentleman who truly made the experience as pleasant as it could be for me. He had a way about him that made me feel like I was the most important person there. I know he made everyone he encountered feel that way. He was just one of those people. He would greet people at the front desk with the best smile and positive energy like rays of sunshine beating down on my face, and it felt like it wrapped around me like a cozy blanket as soon as I walked in. Many times, he would come out from behind the counter to hug Hank and me and ask how we were doing. The great thing is he seemed to do this for everyone.

Despite the jokes, the support, and the love, chemo appointments were excruciating for me. Hank would come to the office to pick me up for a quick lunch and then it was off to chemo. I would drag my feet and do anything and everything I could to keep busy at work. By the time we were ready for our next chemo appointment, I was just starting to feel human again, so the thought of being knocked back down and feeling like death once again was not my top choice of a wonderful TGIF! Needless to say, I was the cause of us being late to a few of our treatment appointments.

When I started the chemo the very first time, I could feel and see this picture in my mind's eye of what was happening inside my body. I can still remember it vividly. It was like something was being poured into my stomach. It started at the bottom and began crawling up or filling up. I could feel it; I could feel it rising up. It was almost like they were pouring something directly into my stomach and I could feel my stomach expanding—but you don't feel like that when you eat! It's almost like when you've had too much water and it's sloshy. It reminded me of the scene in the movie, *The Sixth Sense.* You know the scene where the boy watched the videotape and saw the poor little girl drinking some kind of chemical to clean drain pipes mixed in her soup? Just getting sicker and sicker. Yeah, well, that was how it felt.

My skin turned pale shades of green. I could smell the chemicals from inside me and cleansers all around the treatment area. As the feeling in my stomach grew, everything in my stomach came up; I could feel it rising into my throat. The nausea was growing rapidly. My heart was beating so loudly. I could feel this uncomfortable warmth overwhelming me—and it was scary. It was like, *Ah, hang on. What's going on?!* I remember crying and looking into Hank's eyes and saying, "Honey, I'm so sorry."

"For what?" he asked.

And I said, "I had no idea. I had no idea what you were going through."

That was when he started to cry. And I said, "Now I know. Now I've walked in those shoes." I said that many times throughout my treatment with each new stage and each new side effect. As a caregiver, I thought I understood so much of what he was going through. Unfortunately, I hadn't a clue until then. The only way I can think to describe this pain is about five times the worst flu one could ever imagine.

The sadness that welled up inside me at this time was huge. I could not even imagine a human being going through so much pain. It felt as if I was being poisoned from the inside out. I felt horrible pain both emotionally and physically throughout the whole treatment process. I would never wish this on anyone, but I know this process is what made me so strong today. This is why I am able to help so many people in this lifetime. I am a warrior.

Message from
the Host of Angels

Beloved ones, we are here with you. We are encouraging you to watch the positive mind . . . Watch the negative mind . . .

Be aware that what you bring into your reality will be your experience in this play. Everything is happening in divine order. We ask that you pull back and look from an angelic point of view—to see from a higher perspective what you are going through even though it might feel as though it could not be any worse. We ask you to look at it from a new perspective: look past the intensities that you are experiencing so you can see . . . a bigger picture.

We encourage you, as Stacie has mentioned, to stay positive. Positive affirmations are very much encouraged to keep your spirits high. It is so easy to slip into a low-vibrational frequency when we are focused on all the lower frequencies. Just asking you to surrender the negative thinking, you have control over your thoughts, so as these negative thoughts encroach into your mind, release them. Ask your angels, ask God, ask your team—as Stacie says, your spirit team—to release these negative things that are lying on the surface. Say thank you, but no thank you, and quickly get back on top of the spiral by using positive affirmations. By creating the reality you desire. Speak it as if it has already happened. Speak truth into it. Speak life into it. This shall help your experience.

We are also here as a collective, but we want to remind you that you can call on us specifically for specific needs. You can call on Archangel Raguel for help with these positive affirmations—of these powerful ways of looking at your situation, your reality, to bring in speed to have a resolution quicker.

You can call on Archangel Raphael to bring about healing in a quicker way to manifest that in a quicker, more positive style. But again, we want to remind you that everything happens in divine order, so have faith, dear ones. We have never left you, we will never leave you, we are beside you, we are around you, we are with you. Call us any time you are wanting us to help. You must ask.

And so it is.

Chapter Seven

Inside Out

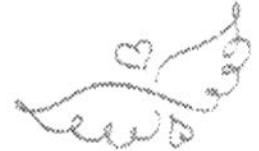

The little kids didn't understand as much, but we talked about it. They didn't have much of an awareness of what was happening and continued going on with their lives, without knowledge of the cancer diagnosis. In a way, this made things easier as they were not attached to the outcome of the situation. We told them, "Mommy might get sick like daddy does," and "I'm gonna lose my hair." Just things like that. My fifteen-year-old understood it more, she was older.

> *Alex, my daughter mentioned in an interview for WVCI's blog, "I really got the concept of cancer when my mom got it. When she was diagnosed,*

that's when I understood, okay, this is really serious."

I think it really scared her—the thought of being without a mom is very scary to a child. She really stepped up during my battle and really helped a lot with our other two little girls. She helped with her little sisters wherever she could. She made food like macaroni and cheese. Got them cereal. Things like that. She was just a kid herself at the time, and didn't really know at first what she was doing or how to take care of someone, so they watched a lot of TV. But she figured it out quickly. She really stepped up to the plate and took an adult role so fast. She blew me away. I know that is hard for a fifteen-year-old child, but I could not have made it without her.

There were days when I was in bed all day, and Alex was my saving grace. She is one of my angels and one of my proudest accomplishments in life. It is funny how having a child makes everything seem all worth it here on earth. I am so grateful for Alex and what she has done for me.

We tried to keep a sense of family as much as possible. Hank set up surround sound in our master bedroom so we could have family movie nights in bed. We tried to focus a lot of the family activities in our bedroom because we just didn't have the strength to go downstairs. We wound up getting a small fridge and a microwave and all kinds of things in the bedroom for those times when we just couldn't function. Neither of us could even go downstairs to the kitchen without extreme fatigue hitting us. And then we didn't know if we would be able to tackle the nineteen steps back up.

It was even scarier to think about when I was home alone. I am not sure how Hank did it, but most of the time he returned to work on Monday morning after chemo on Friday. I was never able to return until Tuesday and sometimes not till Wednesday. When I was done with the treatment completely, I added up all the days I lost to being in bed—maybe it was the OCD side of me kicking in. I figured I probably lost about three months of my life to bed rest in a two-year span. It is probably why today I hate lying in bed for hours on end. Don't get me wrong, I love to sleep till I naturally wake up. However, I now have this antsy, panicky feeling whenever I try to lie in bed all day and be lazy. It drives me absolutely crazy.

There were times both Hank and I would feel great for a day, and then we'd go to do something and just hit a wall. Suddenly there was just no more energy. When I was doing chemo, it was like a light switch—I would be just fine and then the light switch would turn off and I was done! One day, I decided to take my daughter school-clothes shopping with her friend. We drove to a mall. We walked halfway down the mall and that light switch went off, and I was done. I didn't know how I was going to get the girls back home. My poor daughter had to go find a security guard to get a wheelchair. And to think, I even used to tell myself I would never be in a wheelchair. No way! I was Superwoman. I could do it all. But now, suddenly, I couldn't. That day, my daughter had to wheel me around that mall until I had the strength to drive us back home. It was truly a humbling experience.

During this time, I needed to accept that I needed help in my daily life. This was really difficult for me as I wanted to be the superhuman person who could do it all. I had to surrender to the fact my body was not functioning well. This made me rely on my husband and children, which was one of the hardest things in my life. As a mom, it is so hard not to be able to take care of your children the way you envision it should be done.

My own mom was struggling in her own way with my cancer. My family lived in another state and Mom couldn't always be here for everything. That was really hard for her. Mom came to just about all my surgeries and stayed as long as she could while

Dad worked. She is another one of my angels! Everyone has his or her different strengths. One of my mom's is she knows how to be a fabulous, motherly, caring individual (to everyone, not just me). She never forgets special dates and always knows exactly when you need a word of encouragement. She makes everyone around feel included and loved and lets you cry on her shoulder anytime, even if it is only through the phone. There was a time I was feeling so down, and my mom sent a poem to me—a poem that helped strengthen and made me feel a lot better.

I want to share that poem with you now.

Stacie From The Inside-Out

Written By Viki Gardner ©2009

Life is wonderful, without much strife.

A working mother, a loving wife. No time for an extra ride in life.

Who's this person you're talking of? I'm so young, and so in love...

It can't be me, can't you see? I've things to do and places to be.

Wait – slow down, did I hear you say? There is cancer – we can't delay,

My head is confused, don't tell me this, I don't want figures of what – what if...

My world is spinning, crying out – inside,

No, my life – untied! Oh, where can I hide?

I don't want this ride; I can't take this ride!
I'm so young, full of life, with much to do, you see;

One surgery maybe two, maybe three;

Taking away bits and pieces and parts of me...

From the mirror I try to hide;

To the shower, I slip inside,

And cried and cried, and cried......

I don't want this ride; I can't take this ride;

Oh where, oh where can I hide?

Some stare, but others say, "I look fine!"

They see me only part of the time. I don't mind. I know they're being kind.

I'm hiding the aches and pains deep inside; I don't like this ride; I don't want this ride!

There's poking and prodding and chemicals abound;

I'm ill, I'm sick except for the sound — Of loved ones saying, "you're strong – you'll get thru this;" Their encouragement tries to conceal the stress.

My head is spinning; I'm crying inside; I don't WANT this ride; I can't take this ride!

Dear God How Can This Be Fair?! Lying in silent repose – upon the pillow; "my hair."

With lack of hope, I'm grieving – the loss of Me. Who I am and what others see,

Nothing's the same, in utter despair – How can I endure their stares?

Where is the reward for the illness I feel? I keep going back, it seems so uphill.

Till I see their little smiles and voices say, "We need you, Mommy, and when can you play?"

So I'm taking this ride however far or wide; 'Cause I'm loved, not just outside, but on the inside!

I'm taking this ride; — I'm taking this ride!

I went from wearing a size 10 to a small 8 in about one month. I do not recall ever wearing a small in anything! My collar bones started sticking out, and for the first time in my life, my stomach went in instead of out! I felt weak, gross, and like a different person. I had a hard time looking at myself in the mirror as I had changed so much. Ironically, being this skinny was something I had wished for all my life. The days following chemo always felt to me like what I thought nearly dying would be. When I was first diagnosed and they told me I had cancer, I couldn't feel it. But after chemotherapy, I felt like I was dying. Every time. It was as if I was burning from the inside out and could not do anything—get out of bed, make food, or take care of myself.

One day, I was having a really tough day by myself at home in bed. My mom was on the phone with me, and I could hardly hold the phone to my face. I was crying but trying desperately not to cry hard because it hurt too much to cry. My sternum throbbed and ached as well as the bones in my legs. It felt like the bones were imploding on themselves. I had to have a shot of a drug called *Neulasta* the day after chemo to help increase my white blood cell count which, in turn, helps to fight off infection. But the side effect for me was what they called 'bone pain.' This caused my inability to walk due to the heels of my feet and legs being in such pain. I had to crawl to the bathroom during those times. I also had yet to find any food that I could actually eat and keep down.

This is when I felt the weakest. I was barely a person anymore—or at least that was how I viewed things at that time. This is when I felt my life was shattered and all was lost. I still, to this day, do not know how I made it through this phase of my life. I remember the pain and torture I went through so vividly. I would not wish this pain on anyone.

On one particular day, I felt like I was starving to death. Not the kind of starving we get when it's dinnertime and we haven't eaten since breakfast. But the kind of *I hadn't eaten in three damn days*, starving! I hadn't eaten because I couldn't—due to chemotherapy. Then, suddenly, my body felt ready to eat, but I didn't have the strength to hop up and prepare a bunch of food. I told all this to my mom, and I could feel her holding back from crying. I could feel the heaviness in her heart as if she was right there next to me. Dad's tough tom-girl wasn't so tough today. I think my mom called my husband at work after we hung up the phone. He must have called friends and literally had people coming to the house as quickly as they could, some bringing food, some preparing it when they got here. Hank would have come himself, but we didn't live in the same town we worked in. Having such a commute each day, he couldn't personally run home and check on me.

Hank was always so great in these situations. Without even telling me, he got the help I needed at the perfect time. I had so much support surrounding me each day. I am so pleased with how everything turned out; I had angels surrounding me at all times.

One girlfriend arrived and made me fried eggs, grits, pasta; all these weird random things. Then she came upstairs holding out this tray filled with tons of obscure foods, and she said, "Whatever you want, here it is—there's watermelon, there's pasta, eggs . . ."

"Oh, thank you!" I blurted out. This was exactly what I needed because I hadn't figured out what I could eat and what I could hold down. Not to mention there was no way I could make it downstairs.

My friend Cheri mentioned in her interview for the WVCI blog, "As a friend of someone going through cancer themselves, being there for them, watching out for them . . . Ya know, knowing that we could help get her through it just by being there and supporting her . . . "

We had an amazing network of friends that made sure we had dinner for our children and our family every night we were in our worst shape. We would arrive home from chemo Fridays and there would be a hot dinner for our children delivered by our friends. More of my angels!

Alex even mentioned how nice it was to have a lot of people coming to help with the cooking and cleaning. We were very blessed by so many people in our community who stepped up to help. It was not easy for me to receive all this kindness and love. I will never forget a friend telling me how important it was for him and his family to bring us dinner. It was their way of helping—they could make a difference—and that I needed to allow them to do so because allowing them to give was also a blessing for them.

When we learn to receive, we can finally learn to give. Angels have been helping me my whole life and since my cancer treatment, I have finally been able to receive their help. When I learned to receive as a mom and woman, my life changed. I have been a giver my whole life and now I can finally receive from God! THANK YOU!

The Day I Lost My Hair

This was one of the most monumental moments for me throughout the entire process. It was particularly scary because, for some reason, I thought to myself the whole time, *Oh, I'm gonna beat the odds, I'm not gonna lose my hair. Psh, whatever, ya know. I'm different. Ha, ha, whatever.*

Dr. Monticelli said that on the thirteenth day, breast cancer patients generally start losing their hair. So I got to the thirteenth day, and I was like, *I'm golden! This is good – piece-a-cake. I'm gonna keep my long eighties hair and I'm all good.*

Well, I got to work, and I was sitting at my desk, and I felt little things falling on me . . .

So I looked . . . and . . .

Oh, my goodness—chunks of my hair!

I cleaned up those chunks at lightning speed. And then, a little later, more chunks started coming out. These chunks were much bigger. I started to panic. I kept trying to tell myself, *Well, it's just going to thin. It's just going to thin. It'll be okay.*

> *Alex said, "My mom always had to look really, really good. Do her hair, do her make-up every morning. Take like an hour to do it. When she started chemo and she started losing her hair, it was very emotional – very hard to deal with because it was something she valued."*

This was one of the hardest parts of the chemo-treatment for me. I had been attached to my hair and make-up, to feeling "put together." Looking back, I realize how much I identified with my physical beauty. It was important to me. When it was taken away, I felt I was losing myself in this process. I spent a lot of time crying about it, but there was nothing I could do.

My hair thinned all weekend. Monday, when my husband went to work, I woke up with hair all over my pillow. By the time my family got home that night, I just had a few patches left. They left me in the morning looking like Mom and when they got home, I didn't look like Mom. I cried. We had a husband-and-wife moment in the room together and we decided that this was going to be a family event. We were going to have a head-shaving party.

Everybody came into the master bath, lathered up Mom's head and shaved. Everybody got to touch it, kiss it, joke about it, make mini-me jokes—every kind of joke you could imagine. It was like, *Okay, let's just get it all out. C'mon!*

> *Alex said sometime later, "When they decided to shave it, I was kind of shocked, but we ended up shaving it – taking pictures. Letting everybody put the shaving cream on there and just kind of letting everybody have a turn. So it was pretty fun."*

This was a special experience for me. My family always came together to help support me. When we have a ritual or party around a change in our lives, it brings peace to the process. This way there is a milestone marker in our life experience, and we can process the emotions in a healthy way.

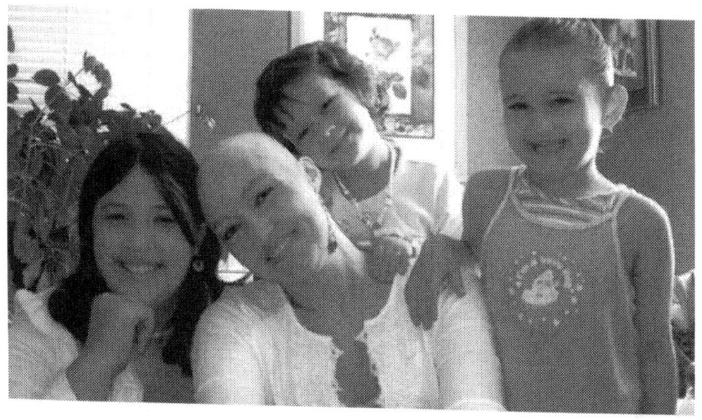

I was comfortable in my home that way. It was weird because before I lost my hair, I *did* panic, and I made a special trip to get a wig that looked almost identical to my own hair. I did wear the wig three times. One day, I had a hot flash while I was wearing the wig in a work meeting, and I felt like I was going to spontaneously combust at any moment. I could not think. It was a very important meeting, and I was itching and moving and trying not to move my hair like this or like that. Finally, I interrupted the meeting.

I said, "I'm so sorry. I just can't take it anymore. I don't want anybody to be shocked. I don't want to offend anybody, but Sophie's gotta go." And I just grabbed the wig and threw it in my desk drawer. The reactions were hilarious! They were all like, *Oh my god! What the heck is she doing!?* They didn't know what to do.

"Oh, thank you! I can concentrate now!" I smiled and got right back to what I was doing. From that day forward, I never wore my wig again—well, except for Halloween.

My friend, Cheri Kistner, said, "I think the thing that's most marked for me about meeting her was how bold she was about that. She just chose to be Stacie. I think that's what we love most about her, that she's just always been right there, wide open."

I have always wanted to stand up and own whatever was happening in my life. This way I could be myself—be open and honest with everyone. When we are able to be vulnerable in the world we allow others to do the same. By taking off my wig and owning my cancer, I believe this helped me to fight! Had I decided to hide it, I wouldn't have been expressing my true self or standing up and stepping out in the way I wanted to. The way I knew I could.

And the nice thing, too, was that my dad called it my badge of honor. And in a way, it was. I was in a position at work where I marketed to different companies, so I would go to these companies and walk around. Now, walking around bald in public is quite an experience. You get all kinds of reactions.

But mostly, I think it was inspiring to other people. And that was my hope. *If I can do this, you can do this.*

I have learned from my cancer experience to be bold and put myself out there. When you are in hiding, due to the fear of embarrassment, you can not hold your own light. As my angels have said, you need to shine your light bright. I think having cancer helped me do that. When we go through an experience like this our light shines brighter afterward. I am so glad I had the courage to be my bold self! I hope this helped others do the same.

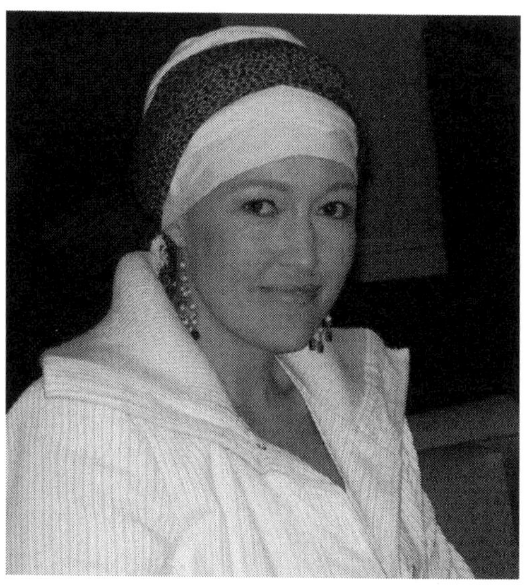

Going through chemo was an interesting journey. If you are one of the beautiful souls out there who has to experience chemo, and you can bring someone with you, do so. Never go alone—I highly, highly, highly recommend you have someone sit next to you during every chemo appointment. And even if it is not for the entire appointment, at least someone should still sit with you for a little while. Because there is a lot of mental stuff going on inside your head, and when you sit there by yourself, you get overwhelmed which can start to mess with you. My husband and I were always the 'glass half-full' kind of people. Once in a while, one or the other would have a low period and the other one would bring us back up to where we were supposed to be.

Many of us think we are weak if we need someone else's help. I know I have said this before, but the more help we receive from others, the more we give to them. Angels in the world want to help us, and if we are too stubborn to ask, we do not get to fully embody the gift of giving. The more help we accept from others and our angels, the more we can give to this world.

One of the nurses said something so great and very important to me. I didn't like hearing it, but it needed to be said, and now I appreciate it. She sat me in my chemo chair and got right in my face. She said, "Stacie, your number one job is saving your life.

So to be on time for your appointment is very important!"

As I mentioned previously, I dragged my feet when it came time for my appointments. I was late a *lot.* The nurse wasn't mad at me; she was just waking me up. I did not like it. In fact, I sat with my knees up in my chair that day, a blanket wrapped around me. I hid my face and cried under that blanket. I was mad because I had to do this whether I wanted to or not. But she was right—getting better was my number one job. I was worried about my career, my job that I had to go to every day. But really, that stuff doesn't matter if you don't survive. So look at doing your treatments as your number one JOB to save your life—I highly recommend it.

We forget this in our lives in general. We value our work and money over our health and family. But having cancer taught me that my health and family is always the most important thing. Without that we have nothing.

Hank and I both believed that everything happens for a reason. We believed in our team of doctors. We believed they wouldn't steer us wrong. Believing in the fact that they had everything in their power to give us the best of the best—we believed that. We believed them when they recommended what was going to be the best for us. Knowing that we were in the war together was great. Believing in them and having the faith that they were not going to steer us wrong, and having faith up above was huge—knowing that the Lord is always going to help us get through each day and not give us any more than we can handle.

I believe the angels were working through the nurses, doctors, and other staff in the hospital. Source works through humans to help us through our challenges in life. These doctors were angels in disguise and always said the right thing at the right time. God was always with me and for that, I will be forever grateful . . . THANK YOU!

Message from

the Host of Angels

Greetings, dear ones. We are happy to be here on this blessed day.

As Stacie has shared how very difficult her journey was during this time of her life, we are encouraging each and every one of you who may be going through a very similar situation or similar health crisis to remember that everything happens in the perfect and most Divine timing.

As your human vessels scream out to you about what is in need of healing, remember that these times are like the tide changing to redirect a ship. God will use these times to redirect you on your Soul's journey. Sometimes crises happen, such as Stacie's health crisis, so that you can redirect your Soul ship. We go with this analogy for you, that even in the midst of these tough crises, we've never left you, and we encourage you, dear ones, to look around . . . to pay attention . . .

to see the signs . . . to see the angels—the Earth Angels who have been placed in your life as Stacie has seen and witnessed firsthand.

We ask you also to look for the light not only within these earth angels, but to look for the light within you. For you, dear one, are a beacon . . . a beacon of light . . . God's light . . . the light within you sparks the light in others. And as Stacie was so brave to share her journey—her crises—with the world, her light sparked others—many others, and those others . . . many others, and those others . . . many others.

God uses all things for good. When you are in the midst of your darkness, know that there is still light and, dear ones, we also know that sometimes it feels hopeless. Sometimes you feel like giving up, surrendering, and coming home because you see or feel a lack of God/Source/light, But we assure you, dear ones, the divine is guiding you each step of the way.

We encourage you to take one step at a time.

We will shine the light on each step as you go take that step, dear ones. Take that ride, like Stacie's poem in this chapter mentions. Choose to take the ride. Choose to play in the play. Choose to experience the contrast—the dark, the light, the good, the bad.

Choose to give gratitude to all.

Choose life, dear ones.

You chose life. You chose to come here. You chose to make a difference.

We encourage you to choose this life—to choose the light. We realize that for some, the contrast has to be so great that it turns your ship. It turns you to face the right direction when you have fallen off the course. Redirecting you, dear ones, redirecting.

We realize that no soul wants to experience, as a human, these troubled times. Though we encourage you to remember that you chose to make this difference, that you chose to come here and experience the polarity that this life has to offer.

Be the Earth Angel.

Shine Your Light.

Share your story and come into the fullness—the beauty of the contrast which is God's light.

And so it is.

Chapter Eight
Reconstruction

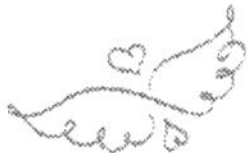

I soon began radiation treatments after chemo was completed. Dr. Julie Gemmell was my doctor at the Willamette Valley Cancer Center. She was such a sweetie. Not old enough to call my 'mom figure,' but more like my 'best-friend' figure. To see her smile despite my fear was very helpful. Just to think—radiation. My gosh! That's scary. What in the world is that? I didn't really know.

Dr. Julie Gemmell was definitely one of my angels. She made me feel at ease and was always caring, kind, and compassionate. Sometimes we think the best doctor is someone who knows the medical field, which is true. Even better is a doctor who knows her stuff and also knows how to make us feel good inside. It makes all the difference.

Dr. Gemmell said, "We had a pretty, bald-headed lady in front of us. When I first met her and Hank, she was very nervous and scared and I could see that. What I talked to Stacie about is how radiation is used in combination with the surgery they've had first. This is in order to gain localized control of the cancer in the breast and the regional lymph nodes. We're different than chemotherapy because chemotherapy is usually administered in an I.V. and it circulates through the whole body, whereas radiation – I like to say it's like shining a flashlight just on one part of your body. I have a lot of shields up inside the top part of my machine and every one of those 80 shields is individually motorized to be placed just exactly where it needs to be to target specific places where the cancer is or was."

When I went in, I kind of felt like a piece of fabric at the fabric store; the way they shuffled me on the table, it was kind of how they shuffle fabric: They line it up, and they keep snipping at it until it's lined up just right. Then they cut it. Well, that's how I felt on the table. I laid there, and they moved the table. Then they lined me up with red lines on the table and left the room. The machine turned on, made a loud noise, and rotated over me. The machine snapped off, the doctors re-entered, and I was all done. It took ten minutes. But then I had to come back the next day. It did make me feel a little bit nauseous at times and sometimes I couldn't eat as well. For the first time in my life, I realized it was a bad thing to lose five pounds in one week. The other symptom I experienced was just being tired. When many of your cells are dying and trying to replicate themselves, there's a lot going on in your body trying to heal. It makes sense that it wore me out.

I became really good friends with the nursing staff there. We shared recipes with each other, always hugged, and Julie was always a beaming light to see every time we were there. I think radiation was a piece of cake compared to chemo. It didn't hurt that I adored the staff.

When looking for a place to get radiation treatment, make sure you enjoy the staff, environment, and trust your gut. When getting treatment, the environment you are in is so important. This will make you *want* to go to the treatments. Your mindset in treatment is as important as what you do while you're there. I learned (and now teach) that what you focus on you get more of. So focusing on those cancer cells being annihilated with every zap was my full intention.

Dr. Gemmel also said this, "Radiation is usually the last stop on the journey – people are starting to feel pretty close to the goal, but they're also feeling pretty worn-out and tired. Stacie had a whole family that she was taking care of. She was a young healthy woman when she came into this whole thing. Taking care of your cancer and your family means that a lot of energy is going out in a lot of directions. Usually, radiation is the part of treatment where your body starts to recover from the chemotherapy. However, in Stacie's case, the chemo was still going on, which meant she was fighting two battles at the same time. But every day in was one day closer to being done."

Reconstruction surgery was the next step, but I had to completely heal from radiation and chemo to give my body time to figure out what the norm was going to be again. I felt like I had been going to doctors forever. There were so many steps to the process. This final step was one that felt right for me and for my family.

My reconstruction doctor was Dr. Movassaghi. He was an amazing perfectionist. I have to say I was pretty scared of reconstruction surgery. We discussed what would look right for me. Being classy was very important. I didn't want it to look like one day I came to work looking normal and the next day I came to work . . . vavoom! I just wanted it to be a nice transition. And so again, my goal was to look good in clothes.

Whether or not to do reconstructive surgery can be a difficult choice. As a woman, I have been told if we get breast implants we think our bodies are not good enough, which is something we struggle with anyway. I was very conflicted between wanting to look great and being modest. Also, I frequently thought about the embarrassment that would come to my family if I got my new breasts that were too large. However, in the end, I made the choice that I felt was best for me.

We started with the first reconstruction surgery. We chose to remove the skin and muscle from my back, weave it under my armpit, and place it all onto my left breast area. There was the option to go from my stomach, but my husband and I still hoped for the option to have a baby and chose not to go this route. When making these decisions it is best to keep your options open and not take risks that could ruin things that might be in your future best interest. During this first surgery, they placed the expander in the reconstructed breast. An expander is just what it sounds like—a contraption that allows the tissue they've placed in your breast to expand. Then, every week when I would go into the office, they would put a needle in the breast area and squeeze in fluid. This would increase the size of the breast, stretching the skin and muscles so it could accommodate the new implants that would be inserted. When this process was complete, I had another surgery so they could remove the expanders and put the implants in.

My surgeons did everything possible to try to save the nipple. But at this point, Dr. Movassaghi said he didn't know if he could still save it. I felt a little discouraged. It had been a lot of trouble to try and save it and I had already been through so much. However, I trusted in my angels and the plan they had for me.

I realized that I might wake up and have to get one tattooed on, which I was fine with. But when I woke up from surgery, it was so funny, because he was trying to pull down the little wrap he had placed on me, and he announced in his distinct accent, "Say hellooooo to your nipple!"

I was truly exhilarated and the doctor was hilarious at just the right moment. I started laughing through the pain, thrilled that he was able to save it. The whole process was phenomenal. I am grateful I trusted the plan of my angels and went through with the procedure despite the hardship and the risk of losing my nipple. Overall, my reconstructive surgery was a success.

After reconstruction surgery, I had to check in with the doctors on a six-month basis to get bloodwork and mammograms done. Those doctors were still a big part of my life: the surgeon, oncologist, nurses, and staff. But things were looking good. I thought we'd won. I was back on my feet after an almost two-year battle. I believe that, during that time, my angels were always there for me and that God was looking out for my best interest. I didn't even realize to what extent my heavenly angels supported me at the time because I didn't communicate with them back then the way I do now. My earthly angels were always on my side, too, and I was able to make it through due to all the support I received during this time. I am thankful for all those—heavenly and earthly—who were looking out of me.

As I felt my body was being reconstructed, Hank's seemed to be giving out more and more. Just when it seemed everything might be all right, just when it seemed we could shake off this cancer and get our lives back, just when we thought our family would be whole again, Hank's condition went in the opposite direction. He was getting sicker and the cancer was growing more. The chemotherapies stopped. We tried experimental things, opening our minds to anything and everything possible. We sought out alternative doctors and researched all the treatments we could.

Hank's life for the last several years had been filled with chemotherapy sessions. He'd gone through it four different times. I couldn't believe how strong he was. I went through it ONCE. And after I did, I told myself that if I ever had to do this again, I would say no. I would just rock 'n roll my way right on out of this world—just live it up and love every moment I had. Chemotherapy was that hard—hard enough that some people choose to die instead of going through it again.

When it came to the time they told Hank he needed to do chemo again—and I was in that doctor's room with them—I welled up with tears. Inside, my selfish side, I said, *You have to do chemo again? You have to be here for us.* But then the other side of me, that side that knew what chemo was like, said—*But I don't blame him if he says, no way. I absolutely don't blame him.* I knew I couldn't make that decision for him. It had to be his decision, and I would support him 110 percent, either way.

He said, "When do we start?" And I just cried. He was a strong man. He did whatever it took. I'm very proud that he did multiple chemo sessions because it's *not* easy. Hank was one of the bravest men I had ever met. He was a great father, husband, and true light warrior. I was so grateful and honored to be his wife.

Message from

Archangel Ariel

Beloved ones, Archangel Ariel is here to share with you the insights in helping you with miracles happening on Earth. In this instance, Stacie shares that the roles were reversed and that her loved one had to make choices in life.

We see that many times we make choices as a human in selfish regards. And as we see in Stacie's journey that Hank made a choice that would benefit his children—a selfless one.

We were there for him. We were there for their family. We were always there. But it was the children who needed the extra time, and he knew he needed to be here longer and was willing and ready to continue to try.

This is the same with God's love—the love for you, beloveds. God would do anything possible for his children.

Many times in life, as a human experiencing the human vessel on Earth, there comes a time when you simply need to surrender to being still.

Not acting out.

Just breathe.

Focus on your own power within.

There comes a time when you can call upon angels. All of us, as your spirit team (as Stacie calls us: her team). There comes a point where there can be healing done on an emotional level—on a spiritual level—which can help on a physical level. But there comes a time when the vessel can no longer be healed at a level it can continue to go.

And this is the time, beloveds . . . It is time to surrender to just being. Non-action. Stillness. Enjoying the miracle of the time you have with your loved ones here on this earth.

Many souls having a human experience on Earth cry out to angels. Cry out to God for healing when the body has gone through so much. And they may cry out wondering why sparing of this life did not or could not happen.

Beloveds, we remind you the vessel is just temporary. Your soul lives on. Your soul just transforms into a different perspective. Many of you grieve the loss of a loved one. We say to you: heal, dear ones. Allow yourself time to heal but know they have never left you. They are right there. We are there. We are right there. God is right there. We are all one.

We see that for souls having a human experience going through these trying times of sickness, of tragedy, of accidents, of times where the body has been pressed and cannot be pressed any further, how hard it is, how difficult it is. And we want you to know, beloveds, there is even more divine love poured out for you at this moment.

The veil tends to be even thinner and your closeness to God is even more.

We are all there, but the hurt of the struggle is so painful that you cannot feel us.

We are like a butterfly wing against your cheek . . . causing you to turn your head.

We are like the whisper in your hair . . . causing you to turn your head.

We are there, beloveds. Feel our embrace. Feel our love.

We are always there.

Sending you love, sending you light, loving you greatly, beloveds.

And so it is.

Chapter Nine

Making Final Dreams Come True

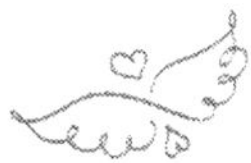

In August of 2009, my oncologist nurse came on her day off to the hospital and pulled me and my husband's best friend aside. She did this to let us know they felt Hank had two weeks left and explained to me everything to expect, what was going on, what they were going to tell Hank. Needless to say, I cried a lot. But I got it all out in the hallway so that I could be strong for my husband.

Hearing this news was one of the hardest moments of my life. I think it may have been even harder than when I found out I had cancer. Hank and I had been through so much, and now I was losing him. What was I going to do? I knew I had to be strong for Hank during his time of transition.

Later that day, I pulled myself together and was able to go back in and be that cheerleader I needed to be for him, because . . . 'Glass half full!' It was our mantra. There is always another way to look at things. There was always light in Hank's eyes.

Susan Coven, the nurse said, "I came in behind the doctors and said, 'Now that they've given you this news, what can we do to make these last few days, months, year, as good as we can?'"

Hank was always a fighter, and I loved that about him. I wanted him to enjoy his time on Earth to the best of our abilities. I loved Hank, and I wanted to be there for him as a positive light, as he had been for me. I adored Hank so much!

Dr. Monticelli told him, "Go have fun. Do whatever you want to do."

Hank thought, *Well, there's another round of chemo we could do.* Dr. Monticelli told him he would do that, definitely. If that's what he wanted to do, that's what he would do. Whatever Hank wanted.

Dr. Monticelli said, "I always tell patients that even if the final outcome is written in stone, we still control how things unfold and the manner in which we deal with it. I think Hank really took that to heart and did as much as he could with a bad situation."

Susan Coven: "He had a type of cancer that would have given him, at diagnosis, a very short time to live, but Dr. Monticelli worked very hard with a lot of other people here in the United States, looking at studies. We tried a lot of really innovative treatments with him."

That night, in the hospital room, I wrote the bucket list. I said, "Honey, what do you want to do?"

"I want to walk on that hot, sunny beach," he told me.

"Great! What else do you want to do?"

"I want to drive that Dodge Charger I had when I was in high school."

"Great. Got it. What else?"

"I want to have a BIG party with all my friends and family."

So I wrote it down: *Celebration of Life*, that was exactly what I wrote down. I wrote down all the things he wanted to do with the kids—the party and family pictures and family time. Knowing what I knew—that he might have two weeks—I then began the craziness of making everything on that list happen for him.

Fulfilling Hank's bucket list became my new purpose and drive in life. I asked myself, "How could I make his time on Earth as fun and joyful as possible?" I became obsessed with how to make his dreams come true and be a positive light in his life. I set myself aside to be there for him during his remaining time on our beautiful planet.

> *Susan Coven: Quality of life played into his whole treatment. The last two years of his life were all based around quality of life. Was he going to have enough time with his children? How could we make a better time for him and Stacie? We tried to taper his services, his chemo, and his other treatments to be around what was important to him."*

We were able to go to Hawaii. I don't know how we were able to go. Flights were so expensive! But the day I searched for tickets they were surprisingly affordable. I booked our whole family right then. The cancer center copied almost his entire chart, "This is what you do if anything happens when you're in Hawaii."

Angels were on my side this day. They wanted him to have his last wishes on earth. I believe our angels guide us toward our desires, especially when they are so strong. I believe this is how we were able to get to Hawaii and fulfill Hank's wishes. I am so grateful for the guidance God provided us during our time of need.

Alex: "We planned the trip because we had thought that Hank only had limited time left, so we wanted to take the last family trip. My step-brother, Tommy, was able to get out of Iraq at the time to come and go on a vacation with us."

Susan: "When a patient has a serviceman that is their child or a grandson or something, we make all attempts to work with the Red Cross and their commanding officers to bring that soldier home. At one point, we thought this was going to be the end for Hank. His son, Tommy, was over in Iraq and we contacted the Red Cross and his commanding officer who were able to get him unembedded and brought home. He also had a huge community base down in California where he was from. He wanted to see some of these people so Stacie, I, and rotary put together a Celebration of Life."

We took time off work and time off school to do what was most important. We had a Celebration of Life with over 300 people. The media came and our doctors came and our nurses came. It was a wonderful day! He reclined on a blanket and people came and sat on the blanket with him and just talked to him. We have pictures and pictures and pictures. At the Celebration of Life, there were many phone calls! We had two Dodge Chargers pull up to the party.

During this time, I realized what was most important in my life. I know we understand this in general, but at times of death, it becomes apparent—what really matters. Having my friends over and celebrating Hank's life was such a memorable and healing experience. In many ways, death brings us closest to life.

As soon as he could, Hank took a spin in one of the Chargers. I had forgotten what it's like not to have air-conditioning in a car! It was very warm! But man, he loved it. One of his other loves was Icees. So we drove that Dodge Charger to the nearest 7-Eleven, got Icees, and piled back in. We drove all the way back and he was on cloud nine. The smile on Hank's face made my heart melt. I am so glad we created the perfect day. We celebrated his life instead of being in mourning and sorrow. This made him feel positive and I believe it made his transition into heaven much easier.

Message from

Archangel Chamuel

Beloved ones, we are here with you today. We have Archangel Chamuel who will speak on the behalf of the collective of the host of angels.

We find that in this message, the beauty of the love that is woven all throughout the Journey of this couple—the frequency of love—has created much healing within Stacie's vessel. Her body. Her vehicle. As she focused on love and noticed many divine miracles happening every day, she could accomplish the things she set out to accomplish. With love, all things are possible.

The frequency of love can heal your own vessel, your own body, your own vehicle, if you will. The frequency of love will also manifest beauty, more peace, more love, more joy to enter into your life.

We also want to preface that a soul is eternal. A soul never dies. Even though we experience life and death (as you know it) alongside you, we experience the heartbreak, we experience the feeling of loss with you side by side.

We encourage you to focus not on the loss but on the presence of your loved ones near you, around you, with you. For the soul is eternal, beloveds. The soul never dies.

There is new life. There are new hopes. There are new dreams, new joys that come with the so-called death you experience in this play. There are opportunities to return to the play. There are opportunities to help from the other side. There are opportunities for that soul to help those who are still here in the play, within the earth construct, to grow on all levels. It is at these times we encourage you to allow your imagination—allow your creativity to grow within that imagination.

Stay open to the ideas. Stay open to the feelings. Stay open to the knowing as you begin to experience in these difficult times of the play. We realized in times of death of the Earthly vessel—the Earthly body—that it is a very sensitive time. Sensitive energies and emotions are very heightened, and we encourage you to honor yourself. Honor these feelings. Feel them, embrace them, and focus on the love.

It is in these times that we find that souls experiencing this human life truly begin to focus—or get focused if you will—on what is important. It makes them stop to think—makes them stop to wonder, "Why am I here?" Wonder, "Is this all there is?" Wonder, what else is there to come?" It is these times, when experiencing the contrast in life, that help you to redirect where your life is going. Co-creating the life you truly want and, in some instances, for some Souls, it is a wake-up call. It is a call to action.

Now is the time.

Now I am remembering.

Now I am shedding away the lessons learned in this lifetime. The lessons that have weighed you down, have covered you up; it is now time to shed these blankets. Remove them layer by layer, to find deep down inside, the beautiful light that you are. The light that carries that love vibration, that carries the love to help light the world's light.

We encourage you to be true to yourself. We encourage you to stand in the present moment and be you.

When a loved one is passing and transitioning to the other side—to the oneness—to all that is, it is a time of opportunity. It is an opening for a community to come together and share in that love.

We encourage this to be a celebration, just as it was a celebration of coming into this world—into this play—we encourage a celebration going into the next space. It is a beautiful thing, and every single soul having a human experience will transition to the other side. We promise you this so we encourage and remind you that these souls have not left you; they are near you; they are one with your soul; they are a part of the collective; they are a part of the oneness, and so we encourage you and remind you again to focus on their presence. Focus on the fact that they are now with you forever, just as angelic beings or other beings are.

We have worked with Stacie for many years, though she had no idea. She knew something was around, something was helping her—opening doors, allowing things to flow, and helping with miracles in her life. However, it took her many years to truly grasp that it was us helping her, and we are honored that she reaches out and works with us now on a regular basis. We are honored that she teaches others how to do so as well, but we want each and every one of you know that we are here for you as well.

Feel the love in your heart. Allow yourself to heal. Allow yourself to feel the emotions and begin to remember who you are: a beautiful, divine being.

We send you love and light.

And so it is.

Chapter Ten
Our Superhero

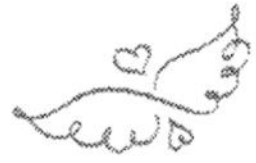

Hank was a superhero to many people—not just us. It wasn't until later in his life that we really started honing in on that Superman thing. We used to joke that chemo was his kryptonite. Every time he got chemo, it knocked him down, but he'd get back up and he'd get back up and he'd get back up.

In the last few months of his life, he wore lots of Superman shirts. And for his last birthday, we had a Superman party. I loved how this honored Hanks' courage and helped him to keep on fighting when things got tough. I believe, as a man, he really was Superman. He saved my life multiple times.

Susan Coven, R.N.: "He loved superheroes and that's why at the end, he had the t-shirt that had the big H on it and the Superman thing."

Dr. Gemmell: "He had a huge fighting spirit. He was not about to give up."

We started going to some counseling with the kids and reading some books, trying to figure out the best way to do this. We knew with my oldest daughter that we had to just talk to her openly like an adult. With our younger ones, it was too hard to understand. So Hank, being really into his superheroes, and the kids always playing Playstation games together, he came up with a story to give them a visualization on how to prepare for this.

He said, "Remember when we used to play those video games?"

"Yeah, Daddy!"

"You know how you get the little pellets, and it gives you life, and your life meter goes up and down?"

"Yeah, yeah, yeah! It's really important that we get that life!"

"Well, you know how sometimes at the end of the game, when you run out of those little life pellets, and you can't find anymore, and your life meter runs out? That's what is happening to Daddy."

And that was how they could understand.

Hank was always so great at explaining things to the children. He was able to connect with them at their level and teach them life lessons in a way they could understand. Watching him do this was a blessing in my life and I felt like he became an angel when connecting with our children.

Dr. Gemmell: "There was no, 'Poor me' attitude. It was just, 'What can you do to help me? Okay, let's go do this!' It was all systems go. Forward. Let's get to the next day because I've got some livin' out there that I wanna do! I want to be here as long as I can."

We spent lots of family time. We would let them have slumber parties in our room. We would have popcorn and movies and do special things like that. This is one of my favorite memories during Hank's transition. It is amazing how the simple times with family are so important in the end.

Susan: "Then we just looked at it on a day-to-day basis. How could we give him the best quality of time with his children so it would be a positive thing at his passing and not be so traumatic and so tragic."

He lived—goodness gracious—a year longer. A whole year! He did do another form of chemo. It was hard. It was really hard on him because he was a lot weaker. Then finally, it was funny, because even when he stopped doing chemo, he felt like he still needed to go to the cancer center every other week, even if it was just to get hydrated. That was his routine—it had been for five and a half years.

"Well, the nurses are waiting for me. They expect me to be there. I need to go there. I need to check in. I need to go do my blood work. I need to go make my rounds and say hello to everyone." That's what he used to say. And so we did that because that's what he needed. Sometimes they didn't know why he was coming. They would ask, "Why don't you just go home and be with your family?" But he needed to do that—they were part of his family. I think going to the hospital every other week made him feel like he was not giving up. If he would have stopped going, I think he would have passed away sooner.

The February before he died, he started to feel worse. A few times, in the middle of the night, he would wake me up and start talking to me. I would have to get up at six in the morning to take the kids to school and go to work. We would wind up talking for a couple of hours in the middle of the night. He'd say, "I think it's time." I would panic, thinking, *Oh my gosh, there's got to be some profound thing I'm supposed to say right now*, but I couldn't say anything. I would just cry.

And then we'd fall asleep and I'd wake up and say, "Should I call into work and tell them I'm not coming?" and he'd say, "No, actually, I feel good now." Aaah! So I felt like we were approaching the abyss and then backing up and coming to the abyss and backing up again. It was a HUGE roller-coaster ride.

> ***Susan Coven, RN: "His end of life came sort of up to that edge a couple of different times, and then we were able to find something new, something a little different and bring him back."***

During this time I felt scared, sad, and confused. I cannot even imagine how my husband was feeling during this process. My emotions were up and down so much of the time. However, I was grateful for Hank's honesty as I always knew what was going on with him. Everything was out in the open. I loved this about him.

Later that month it got really bad, and I took him to the emergency room. They sent us upstairs and checked him into the hospital. He still wasn't willing to give up. He never did give up. He always said, "Oh, there's got to be another solution. There's got to be one more thing, one more thing, one more thing." So we went with it and did it.

Again, Willamette Valley Cancer Center's nurse called me and said, "We think that he has about a week. He'll probably stay the rest of the time at the hospital."

Well, we had already talked, a year ago, about what he wanted, so I became the advocate of making sure it happened. Hank was going to come home.

> ***Susan: "In Hank's case, it was, 'I want to go home and I want to have hydration,' which was a way to help him to extend his life."***

If it wasn't for our friends at the cancer center making it happen, if we hadn't fought to bring him home, we may have had to spend the last few days at the hospital. But instead, we were able to go home and let him be where he wanted to be. All of a sudden he had this spurt of energy. All our family members were there.

This was such a beautiful way for Hank to leave this world. He had exactly what he wanted and the amazing angels around him who helped us get through this process. In a way, it was a celebration of how much we had been through. I was so grateful for all the amazing souls who came there to be present with us at that time, and how they had all affected our lives in different and equally pertinent ways.

On March 1, 2010, he said, "I'm going outside." He had his Superman shirt on and we went outside and sat in the sunshine.

I was like a crazy woman. "Grab the cameras! Get the cameras! Everyone out here! Let's take family photos!"

His best friend from second grade, who had come from California, helped Hank walk up into our tree-house and sit in the tree. The kids sat in the tree limbs and Hank sat in the tree-house—we were all around and we just took fifty photos. Right after the photos were done, the sun moved and wasn't shining there anymore. His energy went down and he went back up to bed.

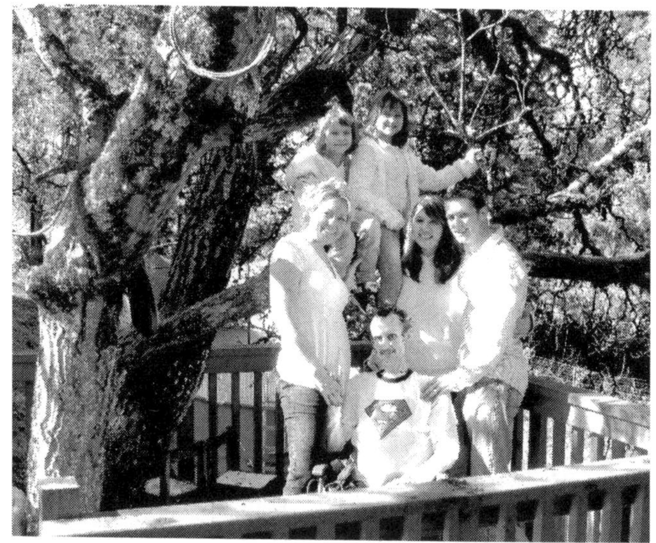

He never left the room from that time on. I had pulled strings to make sure we stayed home till the end. He slipped into a coma for three days before he actually transitioned. The day before that happened, I sat with him in the bed while he napped. In my peripheral, I saw shadows lining our bed. I even looked out the window to see if something was flying by. I have to admit, I freaked out a little. I even emailed the nurse to tell her I thought I was going crazy. She assured me this happens to caregivers sometimes. Strange things can happen around those who are close to death.

There were two angelic presences and three energies I knew to be Hank's loved ones. This was his welcome committee arriving to help Hank transition to heaven. When he woke up, I asked if he had any dreams and he said yes! He was visiting three family members in heaven and they were the same three I had just sensed around him! This was my first experience with the other side. My first communion with angels. Little did I know this was only the beginning for me.

A few days later, right before Hank left to go to the other side, I had a *knowing*, I sat up and looked at him, and I just knew. I started singing and rubbing his stomach. On the third song, the dogs stood up and I felt him move right past me as I kneeled above him. At that time in my journey, I was still not thinking angels, I was thinking "Go to Jesus!"

And he did.

He died in my arms while I sang to him on March 10, 2010.

As heartbreaking as it was, it was such an honor to be by his side during his transition. I felt like angels were helping him cross over to the other side. I am so grateful for God, angels, and the experiences I have gone through in this life. I was so happy and honored to be his wife during this emotional and turbulent time. I am thankful for this every day.

Channeling from

Hank through Debbie

*After writing the foreword for this book, Debbie Motyka sent me this beautiful gift. I knew I had to share it with those who read my story.

He, Hank, came to me over the last few weeks. His energy gently surrounding my space and coming in and out. Today, I asked him if he'd like to share something with me. It was clear he was trying to get my attention, and I had "felt" him around enough now to "know" it was him. There had been times in the past, in which I have lovingly asked a soul, a spirit, for some time, but I knew today, it was the right time to take Hank's words, thoughts, and message and put them on paper. And to share them with you.

He starts by stating the word "soliloquy" with me. So, I asked him what it meant. If he was referring to a play or a type of poem in which one expresses their inner thoughts and self. He said overall, yes (and we agreed I would look it up further to gather the message behind his use of this word). He shares he has been watching you, Stacie, going through your own soliloquy. Almost moving into and through your own deepest inner thoughts and feelings. He shares that it is the most precious, emotional, and moving experience. He is experiencing and helping to assist you from where he is, in heaven, amongst such love and other beloved souls.

God is a part of all beings and processes here, and on Earth, and it's like he's doing this all with Him. But he said your own soul's soliloquy is the reason behind why he is reaching out to me so that I can share this with you.

And in looking up this word, soliloquy, what spoke to me was the description of that of speaking to oneself, relating thoughts, and unspoken reflections. And when one's greatest tragedies can be the way someone wrestles with their private thoughts under pressure, often failing to perceive the flaws in their own thinking—failing to release what is really holding one back.

You have had to examine your own thoughts and your true expression of self. Not just in an emotional, mental, and spiritual way, but also within the methods of writing your book and your works. He says it is like you have been having your own soliloquy which reflects back on your life. It's an inner struggle that has surfaced great confusion, thoughts, pain, and a general feeling of deep emotions, and one that at times feels like a play. A play which you, of course, are a part of, and yet, it has been almost like you have been on the outside looking in.

In this moment of now, you are sitting in the middle of the stage (of your earthly life) and moving through, in, and ultimately expressing aloud your own life's soliloquy. And he has come to help explain to you his thoughts, feelings, and love, about what it is you are going through, in hopes that he may help you, and be able to shed a spotlight on this stage in which you find yourself. He wanted to begin his loving message to you with this word and its meaning and purpose, and I am genuinely and truly hoping that I have done this chosen word, and him, some justice in its explanation to you.

He then shows me a lightning bug. From soliloquy to lightning bugs, but as you know, there is no doubting there is a meaning to it all. So I continue to roll with what and where he is going.

He describes a lightning bug—a firefly full of light and fluttering around, igniting light in the areas among the trees, where it may be dark, and in doing so, illuminates the space and all things around it.

He says you have been like a lightning bug, working so hard at illuminating and expanding light, but have been flying with a broken wing. Not one, which stops your flight, but makes it much more difficult, and at times, even painful for you. This wing was broken, wounded, during your life, in particular from parts of life that you had shared with him, more specifically, from his passing and its aftermath. There was not enough healing, or time for you to really focus on what it—your wing—needed to become whole again.

You were fighting your own battle, and this needed or almost required that you take the safest route in the handling of my loss. In order to keep the energy that you needed for your fight for life, all these emotions, feelings and intensity of our life together needed to be placed into a box with a bow, and safely put away up on a shelf, and it was because of this you were almost frozen in time. You and your beautiful bent and broken wing. And this wing simply became a part of who you are, living with it, as simply an acceptance of the experience of us. Because life had to move on. And your light, albeit, dim at times, almost like Tinkerbell after she drank the poison, you would somehow receive the love you needed, or you'd find the energy required to boost your inner light back to life. Giving you the light to not only exude a spirit and love-filled glow again, but fly despite your broken wing. But yet, this wing, it was bent, somewhat broken, and unable to give you the true lift which you needed to open up and soar without limits.

Being determined, being a survivor, you simply grew to believe that this wing was permanent, and you embraced it as just a part of who you are. You flickered and sprinkled your light, showing the way for others to do the same, giving the darkness a glow for others to see and follow. And when this wing got painful, or you needed to rest, you would manage to stop for a minute (laughing at this...saying "she can only stop for a minute!") to allow it enough rest, and then you'd keep on going. Focusing on igniting the light of others, expanding the light in the darkness, loving and giving yourself to others . . . and I must say, at times, to simply and outright avoid that box with a bow tucked away safely up on the shelf. It was a box you had filled with beautiful notes, music, memories (dancing under the stars), but it was also filled with pain, suffering, and those real and tragic human emotional memories.

You convinced yourself that it was best to remember the good times, honor the glory in the moments that we had spent together. To embrace the love—not explore the pain held tightly within that box. So, you continued to fly—flew on your broken wing. Until now, when you find yourself sitting silently on a branch among the trees. Your light going on and off, you cannot seem to find a way to fly as you had before. It is because you have found yourself in a place in which you have had to open this beautiful box with a bow, and to accept, explore, define, and write your own soliloquy.

Out in center stage, this branch among the trees, feeling quite alone, yet, needing to dig deep into its contents in any hopes to fully fly again. It was filled with so much more than you had remembered, even somewhat different than you had come to believe, and you had even pondered the thought of closing it all back up and putting it away. It was so life-reiterating, allowing you to remember all of it—the good, bad and ugly. For the first time, allowing the real truth and soul pain to become reality. Holding, gripping on tight to the branch so you would not slip off, and really not knowing if you'd fly.

In this space, you felt somewhat weak, vulnerable, and yet, said "I know how to handle this," and, "I am good. I teach this stuff, for God's sake." There was this mental tug of war and pull of your emotions. And I will share, that bringing up weaknesses with you is not something you like to admit or to hear (he is laughing...noting there is such strength of your character, and yet, a sheer stubbornness in your will and drive).

Retelling this story was one of the first times you remembered the true gut-wrenching pain of the end of my life, of our unlived life on Earth, and the secret hole in daily life—that quiet missing spot in your heart I had left. You were allowing it to come forth not really knowing how it would end. I mean, seeing you come forward, hearing your cries, listening to your heart, and how it did knock you off that branch, is why I am here, expressing to you my thoughts.

To the ground you quietly stumbled and sitting now in the grass, your light still flickering, but it just did not seem as bright. "What happened?" you asked. "Why now?" you grudgingly mumbled. "What purpose does this serve at this point in the game?" You know that feeling when you've won the baseball game and don't understand why you are still feeling disappointed? I felt your resistance and the struggle with the emotions of always being and needing to be strong, of being the role model and brave one, and a teacher of teachers.

To fight through these emotions and feelings that were locked tight up inside this beautiful box with a bow was quite inspiring, beautiful, and difficult to watch. But I was there, in and around you, and I believe the feeling of working through this box brought us to a new place, to create a new place for us to exist. A place of peace which you can heal and fix your wing.

I send my love, and I know that you "feel" me, and I see that your light grows a bit brighter and stronger again. Enough for you to fly back up onto your branch of hope. You sit watching your wing begin to heal. It is healing on levels which you did not know even needed such healing and love.

Inside this is the feeling of moving forward into a future that this box with a bow is no longer a part of your life seems to bring about a sense of strange awkwardness and uncertain emotions. What is this you say? It is understanding that I come with you, and I am a part of you, but my human piece in your story is through. You and I served our purpose to each other and we are now a part of one another on a level that even you will not come to fully understand until you are here.

It is okay to throw away this box now. It is of no service to you and what lies ahead. Creating this new space of connection with me, and what this all means, is going to bring about great awareness of self. Of yourself. As I sit, watch you flutter your wings, I see the magic of you. I see you flitter, shine, flicker and are ready for takeoff. This time when you fly it's with full wings and will take you to places you cannot imagine just yet, my love. Treasure this time. Time to heal your wounds and fix your broken wing. Time to take the beautiful box, and open it, and leave it there, where it now belongs. I give you my love, permission if you will, to soar on and light up the skies. I am in you now, not just a part of you. I know you understand this. Carry me through you and not separate from you any longer. There is no separateness in the hereafter. We understand this much more fully than it is humanly possible on earth. But I know that you get what it is I am saying.

Your Larry [referring to Stacie's current husband], I must say, what I truly love about him is that he sees and feels so much of what it is I speak of. Yet, he is not feeling less than or jealous of me (in the human way) but knows and embraces that I am a part of who you are. He does not walk in my shadow, but he lives beside and within it. His love is allowing you the space you need to become all that you are. He loves you with the presence of great unselfishness and commitment. Allowing you to be all you are in the past, present, and future. I admire him in that way. Although it was said, you know how I felt, never feel that in completely letting go, and fully loving Larry, you will not be loving and honoring me. Just a human reminder I felt I needed to say, to share. You know this, of course, I just wanted to say it to you aloud. Larry is a very good man, a gentleman, even though I showed Deb the Beauty and the Beast...I reinforced that I meant Larry is very much a guy/man type and you are like a beauty queen. Almost somewhat opposite, yet perfect, in so many ways. We (Deb and I) shared a laugh over that analogy.

I am working with Archangel Gabriel who has been helping me most as of late. With his green energy of God's true light and love. We enjoy the same fashion sense and humor (laughing). I, too, have had some great growth in such little time. Ah, yes, time and the concept of time here is so different, as you know. My heart light is brighter, too, my love. And we have both brought our heart lights to a much higher place. You are within mine now, literally, and I am within yours. I am learning even more about our Heavenly Father, and Jesus is a miracle all and in Himself to witness.

I am working on writings. The literature and depth of language and understanding have brought about another level of education and writing exploration. My job here is ever forming, certainly not ready to stick to one thing just yet. But you knew how much I loved to read, teasing the mind, utilizing the brain and its knowledge, and now I can take it to the next step of learning and growth, of expansion. But must say I still do love a good book. I hope to expand knowledge here *with my writings one day. I explore more of all that is, and I will continue to watch you fly, my lightning bug, my beautiful firefly. Now with full wings to and from the woods. Lighting up and glowing for all to see. I "see" you and never doubt that your glow is filled with such greatness and healing, but make sure, as you have heard before, that you stop and take care of your heart light once in a while. And for more than a minute, okay?! *Laughing**

Deb's notes: I love the parallels of the soliloquy and the play references. Since Stacie has so often described our earthly life as a play. And at times, needing to take a look at your life in and from the perspective of being the observer. And how the book references, and writings, are also a part of his message as well. So many current connections, so many parallels, and meanings in this, that it makes my own emotions, thoughts, feelings, mind, and soul move. What has brought me to this place in my own spiritual awakening, to reach a moment of compiling such a message, has been because of the love, guidance, and teachings of not only Stacie but now, of and from her Hank. There is a deep soul feeling of him being a teacher, a professor, and his leading me through this writing of such heavenly love has allowed my own spiritual gifts to even further be opened. It is a gift from God, and a true honor, to be able to be a messenger. I thank Our Heavenly Father, and I thank you, Hank, for your trust in me, for guiding me through this piece of love, your love notes to your Stacie. And to Stacie, for giving me such unconditional love, allowing me to learn and grow, both from her beautiful teachings and from shining her heart light on and in my life. I am so blessed and grateful for her continued belief in me and who I AM. It has allowed my heart song to be so much more, to be sung with much more depth, love, and hope. Stacie has genuinely helped me to even further ignite my own inner firefly!!

-Deb

Chapter Eleven

Moving Forward

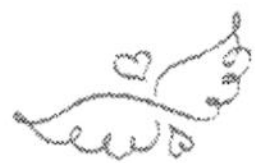

I always have this little visual of God looking down on me and when something in my life is tough or someone is rubbing me the wrong way. I imagine that this is God's sandpaper and He's softening that edge because He's making a masterpiece. And in the end, those things that are tough mold you and make you into a better person and into that masterpiece you're supposed to be.

God is always bringing us miracles even though they are sometimes disguised as adversity or challenge. The obstacles in life help us to shine our light even brighter. Having cancer, losing Hank; all these things were so hard, but they helped me become more loving, caring, and compassionate. Source is always making us stronger, brighter, and more courageous.

We might not have all the answers right now, or understand why we've gone through what we've gone through, but I truly believe that what I've gone through was for a reason. That I'm supposed to help other people. I'm here to be an inspiration and a motivation for others to know that I went through it and so can you. You can do this. I also know that when we experience such intense things in life, it is an opportunity to shift our perception of life. To help us focus on our soul purpose. Why did our soul come to this life? Are we doing what we came here to do? It redirects us and aligns us with that path so we can complete our mission. I believe my cancer was my redirect.

No matter what your trial is, it's like chemo in that it hits you, and it knocks you down, and it knocks you down, and it knocks you down—but you get back up! You keep taking another step. You do what it takes.

Hank taught me never to quit, to always push forward and stay positive no matter what obstacles come along. Some believe God puts these obstacles on our path, but I have come to understand that we actually place them on our own path. This may seem absurd to many, but from a soul-level, we make very different decisions that can be hard for us to imagine in our now-state—our physical state.

Hank used to compare chemo to when he played football. In high school, his team had the smallest football players in their district. No one expected them to win, but their coach told them, "You get back up. You get hit and you get back up and you just keep going for it." They won the state championship that year. Even though they were the underdogs! Teeny-tiny little guys from a small-town country school.

All through his cancer and chemo, Hank believed that he could do what it takes. And he did. So can you—in any situation.

And you do. So many people love you and rely on you: your co-workers, your family, your friends, your daughters, your sons, aunts, and uncles. They need you to be here. Hank felt like his only choice was to keep going and push forward. This is what made Hank so strong.

Sometimes we get wrapped up and feel like the things that happen in life are just about us. But they're not. It's about everyone else around you and everyone else watching you. It's a ripple effect. I didn't realize how impactful my experiences would be. I didn't realize that what I went through would touch so many lives.

When we are not focused on ourselves we find a new level of courage, positivity, and grace. It is as if our service to others is the fuel that keeps us going. It gets us out of the victim role. Instead, we are required to be our best selves to the benefit of all.

Dr. Monticelli: "It's really encouraging to see that she's been able to get back to a relatively normal life, be successful in that life – but also to be able to reach out to others to help pull them through that path and help them get back onto the path back to a normal life. Nobody has a perspective on this like the patients who have experienced it. If there's anybody that can guide somebody through the minefield, it's a former patient."

I've been truly blessed to be able to speak at events and share my stories. I think one of the biggest events I spoke at was 3,000 people. At the time, I still had cancer. I was doing chemo that day—I don't even know what I said, but I had people come up to me with tears in their eyes and thank me. I wished I would have had it on camera because I can't remember what I said. But I was bald, sitting on stage, inspiring others. Obviously, God's used me as a vessel of His love to share exactly what everybody needed to hear that day.

This experience of bringing God's word to people on Earth is called channeling. And everyone can do it in some form. Over the years, it's something I've learned to do more and more. Now I can bring angels' messages through during my life and my work for the benefit of all. I have been able to experience this multiple times in my life and I am now honored to be able to do this for others. I believe our job on this planet is to uplift others in whatever ways we can.

We all affect and touch so many people's lives. And everyone plays a role—whether it's the nurse, or the person who takes your blood, or the receptionist at the front desk—we're all in it together. I am so grateful for the staff and people in my life who have uplifted me during my battle with cancer. THANK YOU! Thank you! Thank you!

Message from
the Host of Angels

We angels are here to share with you today the importance of the maintenance of the vessel this body houses—the Beautiful Soul that you are. This body is what allows you to participate in this Earthly play, and we angels and your spirit team will do everything we can—when asked—to help encourage you and shed light on the directions and the steps you need to take.

We ask you to pay attention to this physical body. Especially when things are repeatedly coming up. This body has been made in a way to allow you to understand and to know if there is a need . . . a need for healing. The body triggers a mechanism that releases understanding to the brain to the outward knowing, and it is time to go within and heal.

It is like any instrument you would play music that needs tending to—it needs to be polished. It needs oil. It needs to be tuned. Your human vessel is the same way. For you to feel terrific and great in this human body, you must treat it properly.

Nourish it with high-vibrational-frequency-type foods. You must exercise. You must work the organs accordingly so that your human vessel will be at the optimal health capacity—so that your soul can fulfill its purpose.

We angels will give you guidance when you ask. You will be rewarded with beautiful energy and happiness. You will even have the motivation to do more things, such as exercise. We also encourage you to spend time outdoors in nature with trees, with the animals, with the wind.

We will help you with cravings, with addictions, we will help you to choose what is better for your body. You have a newfound love that you never knew you loved before. Find a place in your heart to put yourself first. Maintain the utmost, best conducive atmosphere within your own body.

We encourage you to release overthinking, release obsessive thinking, especially when you have a diagnosis—a disease in your body. Turn this over to your angels, to God, and more clarity will come to the situation. When healing the body from disease, we encourage you, dear ones, to focus on healing, focus on rest and repair.

We encourage you not to focus on the despair and the negativity. We encourage you to focus on healing. We also encourage you to go within for emotional healing, for spiritual healing, and ask yourself what this illness is trying to tell you.

Visualize wellness. Visualize diseased cells that are no longer wanted in the body disintegrating. Visualize them disappearing with God's white light. Spend every day doing things that make you feel good. Spend every day finding joy. Finding things in life that bring you happiness. Remember this is about your mission—this is about your Soul's purpose.

Have faith in your team, have faith in your medicine, and have faith that you, dear ones, have the power to heal. Healing is on multiple levels. It is not just on the physical form. Healing must take place in the mind, the body, and the soul. You cannot fix one without the other. Dear ones, you are worthy of healing. You are worthy of great joy. You are worthy of love, dear ones, do not be afraid.

And so it is.

Epilogue

What I Am Doing Now

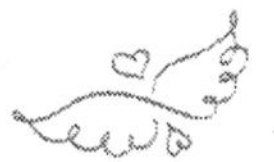

Losing Hank obviously changed everything for me. But it also opened doors I never dreamed of. He is with me still. He comes to me. He reassures me everything is as it needs to be. We still love each other. He even encouraged me (from the other side) to marry my wonderful current husband, Larry. But that is a story for another book.

My life is very different now, and Larry has supported me through all of it (and so has Hank). Because I came from a Christian background, I was torn after my incredible near-death experience. I knew I wanted to be a spiritual teacher because I battled cancer with my husband and even watched as angels showed up around his deathbed.

Before that, I was in church all the time. I spoke there, went to Bible study. Now these experiences I was having were supposedly not okay—of the "dark side" even.

But I knew I wasn't dabbling in the dark side. I also wasn't asking for these things to happen. And although I thought I was crazy at first and didn't know how to explain any of it, I could feel in my heart that it was a spiritual gift. A gift I couldn't ignore.

I started to meet some other sensitives who experienced the same types of things, so I finally had confirmation I wasn't crazy! I worked with a mentor for a bit, and it validated me, but I wanted more—I *needed* more. So I relocated out into the country. In the middle of nowhere, where I felt like a monk on a mountain. I spent all this time alone just painting and sitting in nature. Turning the world off for six whole months. Finally, I realized I was channeling these angel messages through the colors and shapes I painted. That's when I knew I had to practice with other people.

So I started practicing via distance. Phone call, Skype, you name it. And this was extremely successful. This wasn't just for an hour-long reading, oh no, I spent an hour beforehand preparing to hold space for them, writing, channeling, tuning in. I would get on the phone with these people and sometimes just talk for the full sixty minutes without letting them say a word. Then, at the end, when the time was up, I would just blurt out, "Okay, thanks. Bye!" It was weird, but I thought to myself, *Holy cow! Did that just happen?*

The testimonials came pouring in. I was changing people's lives and they were grateful! This was incredible, but it helped me realize I wasn't serving at the highest level because I wasn't giving enough or spending enough time with the client to understand their deepest wounds and needs. I could give them more, and I knew this gift was ready and waiting to expand out of me like a mighty explosion.

I set up my *New You* program to bless lives on an ongoing basis. To heal them so profoundly over time, and not just for hours or days. I needed that kind of involvement to really be what I needed to be for them. These blessed souls who wanted my help.

The universe stepped in and helped everything come together. I'm not doing the work *for* them. I'm giving them the tools to heal on a deep soul level, so they don't have to search out a mentor anymore. So they can serve as light-beings themselves on a high level.

This has allowed me to shift my whole perspective and become a teacher of teachers. I now understand that I am leading the next wave of lightworkers to step up and be leaders themselves.

I *know* I am part of the next wave, and the beautiful souls I work with are the next wave after that, helping others light their lights so brightly they don't even realize they're making a difference. But these souls are healing with every step they take without even saying a word. People just know there is something about them. That's how they are creating a ripple effect, and continuing that ripple effect on and on for eternity. What a gift!

Most people don't understand that the mind, body, and soul are so connected. If they did, they would realize there is an opportunity when the body screams out for help. If they had the tools to heal on an emotional level, the body could heal to a point where they wouldn't be dealing with dis-ease. I genuinely believe if I had the understanding of how to do that back then, I would never have had to battle breast cancer. I would love to prevent dis-ease for others as well.

I am proud to be reigniting the light for these individuals. The lights that had previously been snuffed out. But now, because I have chosen to step out and shine my light, they are sparking their lights once again and getting brighter. I see it every day. My clients look happier and feel lighter and brighter. I am proud to be such a big part of their journeys.

"Now I **WING** it!"

~Stacie

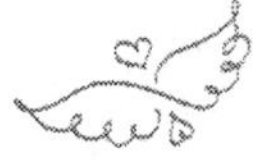

Stacie and her Host of Angels are working wing to wing to help beautiful souls heal on a deep soul level so they can live with more peace, love, and joy. Guiding people through a transformational life change. If you are ready to change your life TODAY, click on the link below to take that first step.

If you are interested in working in the *New You* program, please visit www.stacieoverman.com

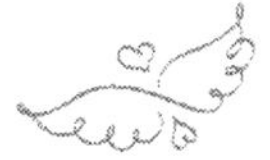

About the Author

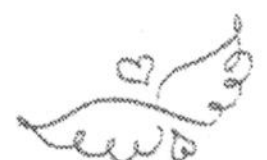

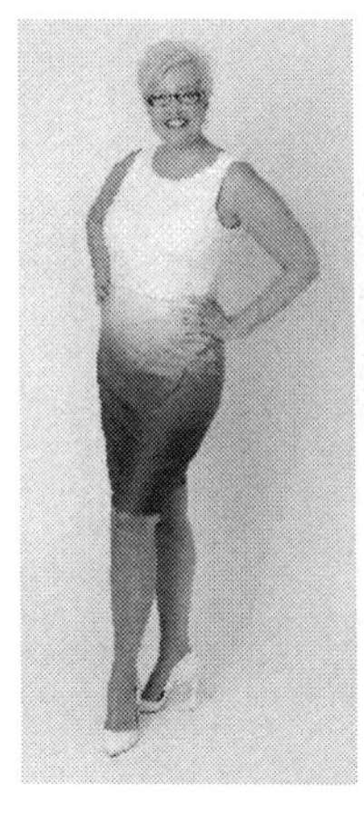

Stacie Overman is a national speaker, spiritual coach, and author who has been guiding clients on a journey of spiritual awakening for over four years.

After surviving cancer in 2006, she found herself connecting directly and beautifully with angels, which led her to write *Angel Kisses No More Cancer*.

Founder of *The New You* coaching program, Stacie's powerful angelic mediumship work has been praised as "nothing short of a miracle" (Henry Jones, Massage Therapy Instructor, Texas Health School).

With a background in entrepreneurship and talent scouting, Stacie was the first spokesmodel for the

Willamette Valley Cancer Institute, where she underwent her cancer treatments in Eugene, Oregon. She made an appearance in the hit series, *Ghost Mine* (SYFY Network).

Stacie enjoys painting angels, travelling by RV with her husband, Larry (vowing to visit every US state before they retire), and spending as much time as possible with her precious family.

Connect with Stacie at stacieoverman.com, as well as in her lively Facebook community *Understanding Divine Messages* where she helps over 7,500 lightworkers connect with spirit, heal, and enlighten the world.

Appendices

MEDIA RELATED TO OUR STORY

Locally filmed 'The Note' tackles cancer issues

Posted: Thursday, Mar 20th, 2008

BY: JOE HANSEN

Sitting in the chapel at Cottage Grove Community Hospital, Hank Sisk, having just lost his daughter to cancer, looked sky-ward with tears in his eyes.

"Why do little children get cancer?" he asked. "Where were you, God, when my daughter needed you?"

Thankfully, this scene was a work of fiction, part of a movie Hank, his wife Stacie and a crew of more than 30 volunteer actors, directors, cameramen, producers and experts are creating about cancer. A portion of the production was filmed at the Cottage Grove Community Hospital March 15.

Cancer is a topic with which Hank and Stacie, of Cottage Grove, are intimately familiar. Stacie recently won a two-year battle with invasive stage 2-breast cancer, having been cancer-free for the past six months.

Hank's struggle is ongoing. In 2003 he was diagnosed with a type of gastrointestinal cancer similar to colon cancer.

"I was originally diagnosed with three to six months of life," said Hank. "Here I am now, five years later."

Hank and Stacie decided to make the movie, called "The Note," in an attempt to raise cancer awareness and money for the Relay for Life, a national cancer benefit relay now held in thou-sands of cities across the nation, including Cottage Grove. The 2007 Cottage Grove Relay for Life raised $55,394 for cancer re-search.

"The Note" deals with a parent's worst nightmare Hank and Stacie lose a young daughter, Haley, to cancer. The idea is based on the couple's own terrifying and trying experiences with cancer treatment.

"It breaks my heart to think of a child going through this, not understanding why they're having to go to this building and feel bad all the time," said Stacie, referring to her own knowledge of what chemotherapy can be like.

After the couple loses their daughter in the film, Hank receives a letter from her, written from beyond the grave, which only he can read to all others, it's a blank piece of paper. This, the basis for the title of the short film, is also inspired by personal experience, as Hank's two daughters are always leaving notes around the house for him.

"The Note" came about through the volunteerism of dozens of people, many of them cancer survivors in their own right, including Director Leonard Henderson.

Rod Butler donated his time as the lead cameraman, for ex-ample, as did makeup artist David Pratt, whose work can be seen in productions such as the films "Men of Honor," "The Haunted," and the television show "America's Most Wanted."

Hank's own oncologist, Dr. Andrew Monticelli, was even on set to offer technical advice about cancer terminology.

The filming of a movie dealing with a topic so close to home amounted to an emotional ordeal for Hank and Stacie, but they said it's worth it to raise awareness with the film, which they plan to show at Eugene Rotary and enter into several film festivals.

"People need to realize that cancer can happen to anyone," said Hank.

But at the end of the day, regardless of the emotional nature of the subject matter, there was still a movie to make, a fact the bustle on the set at Cottage Grove Hospital reflected.

As Hank sat in the chapel at Cottage Grove Community Hospital and asked God why his daughter had to die, the scene cut.

"I love it," said Director Henderson. "Now we're going to do it just once more."

A brief, Timeless Love Story Ends

A couple that shared cancer cherished their five years together

By Mark Baker

The Register-Guard

/.byline

APPEARED IN PRINT: SUNDAY, MARCH 28, 2010, PAGE B1

Theirs was a love story to end all love stories. A love story maybe even "Love Story" couldn't compete with — because Hank and Stacie Sisk's story was true.

Not that they, or their marriage, were perfect. It was her second marriage and his third.

And on the day they were married, Nov. 27, 2004, they knew they might not have much time together.

"We talked about it," Stacie said Saturday after her husband's memorial service at the Eugene Faith Center. "How can you deal with it if I only have three months to live?" Hank asked her in the weeks after proposing.

"We'll deal with it moment by moment, day by day," Stacie told him.

"And I'm so blessed that I had 5-1/2 years," she said. She has no regrets. "We packed memory-making moments in. It's like we were married for 20 years," she said. And, yes, she means that in a good way. "Obviously, I wish we'd had the 20 years, but. …"

But how did Hank Sisk, a multimedia producer, even make it to age 43 after being diagnosed with a rare form of gastrointestinal cancer almost seven years ago? How did he make it to March 13 after Stacie drove him from their Cottage Grove home to the emergency room at Sacred Heart Medical Center at Riverbend on Feb. 7?

"Every time I talked about Hank, my next phrase was: All bets are off with this guy," Jim Jenkins, pastor at the Cottage Grove Faith Center, said during the two-hour service attended by about 200 friends and family members.

The Sisks' story is all the more remarkable when you consider what happened 14 months after their wedding day. On Jan. 25, 2006, 36-year-old Stacie, a personal banker at the Wells Fargo branch in Cottage Grove and owner of her own talent agency, was diagnosed with breast cancer. Hank was by her side through four operations, still battling his own cancer that doctors said would take his life within a year.

They received their chemotherapy treatments in the same chair at the Willamette Valley Cancer Institute. They served as co-ambassadors of the American Cancer Society's annual Relay for Life in 2006.

They participated in the relay every year thereafter, raising about $3,000, Stacie said.

Today, her cancer is 20 months in remission. But she will be there in July when the 2010 Relay for Life kicks off. "I definitely plan on being a part of Relay for Life for life, or until we find a cure," she said.

"Superdad."

John Henry Sisk was born on April 7, 1966, in Las Vegas to Gilford and Nora Sisk, the youngest of three children. His two sisters are both quite a bit older.

"We called him the 'Geritol baby,'" his sister, Vickie Woodcook, said Saturday, after Stacie and her daughter, Alex Henderson, 16, and two step-daughters, Marissa Sisk, 10, and Haley Sisk, 8, had let 50 yellow and green and blue balloons float toward the sky in memory of Hank.

He loved superheroes and comic books as a boy, and Superman was his favorite. To his daughters, and his stepson, Thomas Fotta, now a 23-year-old Army man stationed in Georgia, Hank became known as "Superdad" through his brave battle with cancer.

He was raised in Igo, Calif., an unincorporated community of about 600 west of Redding, where he wore cowboy hats and drove his black 1968 Dodge Charger in high school.

His best friend since fifth grade, Mike Jones, who spoke at the service Saturday, remembered that Hank "had my back" before he even really knew him. And, of course, Hank had his sense of humor. A mean kid challenged Jones, the new boy at school, to a fight one day. Hank showed up and jumped between them at the last second.

"Hold on!" Hank hollered, flashing a piece of paper. Jones thought it might be some sort of "peace treaty." Nope, just an announcement.

"Welcome, everybody, to the big fight between Mike Jones and ..." 10-year-old, freckle-nosed Hank said.

At a funeral, the sound of 200 people laughing is good.

Hank, who worked making TV commercials for Adlib Advertising in Eugene, was already an actor/director at age 12, Jones remembered. They used to roam the creeks around Igo making "war movies," Jones said. Around the seventh or eighth grade, Hank "actually wrote a 15-minute screenplay based on 'Star Wars,'" he said. Hank was Darth Vader and Jones was Obi-Wan Kenobi. But Hank's handwriting wasn't so good. Jones mistook an 'H' for a 'W' and belted out the line, "Weed my word, Darth Vader" as he swung his fake lightsaber.

The two played football together at Shasta High School, Hank wearing no. 44, his favorite number. He went on to play football as a defensive back at Shasta College and graduated from Chico State in 1988.

"Glimmer of hope"

Hank and Stacie met in 1993. They were on opposite softball teams in a Eugene recreation league. A few years later, their teams merged. Hank was the coach of the Emporium Plate Smashers and played second base. Stacie played first base.

During a game in September 2004, after both their marriages had ended, Hank proposed. Stacie was at bat at the Amazon North Field by South Eugene High School. The umpire called her out for wearing jewelry. What jewelry? Suddenly, Hank was on his knees with a ring. She said yes, then belted a home run over the fence.

Hank loved softball. "It could be the bottom of the last inning with two outs, and my father could pull everyone together and give a glimmer of hope," said Fotta, his stepson from his first marriage, in a video recording sent from Georgia that was shown at the memorial service.

A glimmer of hope.

Hank was always giving that, and more, before his deadly diagnosis and after, his family and friends recalled Saturday. "To me, my father was the very definition of strength," Fotta said. "Not because he could lift a million pounds. His strength came from within."

Hank and his fellow Eugene Delta Rotary Club member Tony Metcalf had breakfast one day, and Hank had a question for Metcalf. "What is God's reason for keeping me around?"

"He wants you to spend more time with your friends and family," Metcalf told him. "I never heard Hank complain," Metcalf said during the service. "He never allowed selfishness or bitterness to rule his life. Some would call it grace."

"He died in my arms."

One of Hank's dreams was to make a movie. In 2008, he did just that. It's just a 20-minute film called "The Note," about a family that loses a daughter to cancer. But it was Hank's pride and joy. It's a cancer awareness film starring Hank and Stacie and their three daughters and produced with cancer survivors.

In the movie, the daughter who has died of cancer, portrayed by Haley, writes comforting letters to her father from heaven. The words are invisible to everyone but him. The screenplay is based on the notes Haley wrote to her father in real life during his cancer battle.

After a few days in the hospital in February, Hank returned home to Cottage Grove; to a morphine drip and his own bed. Doctors said he would be lucky to make it through the month. But, as always, he lasted longer than anyone thought he would. "I had a gut feeling he was trying to make it to his 44th birthday," Stacie said, referring to both his favorite number and April 7.

"He died in my arms. He was looking right into my eyes. It was pretty amazing."

It was 5:44 p.m.

Hundreds mourn local cancer spokesman, coach, father

Posted: Tuesday, Mar 30th, 2010

By Jon Stinnett The Cottage Grove Sentinel

Cottage Grove's Hank Sisk lost a protracted battle with a rare form of gastrointestinal cancer on March 13 of this year. But evidence of the lives he touched can be found in many places.

There's "The Note," a 20-minute film about dealing with the effects of cancer that he made with his wife of 5 ½ years, Stacie, herself a cancer survivor. A softball team in Eugene bore the name "Hank's Raiders" during Hanks' cancer fight, in honor of his grit, determination and positive outlook. The Sisks began participating in Relay for Life in 2006, and you'll find Stacie Sisk carrying on in Hank's memory at this year's event in Cottage Grove. Television viewers can still see his work in countless commercials, and the couple's talent agency, Moonlight Talent, put many local acting hopefuls on screen. There are also the support groups, which the Sisks started after Hank repeatedly out-lived the members of groups he had been attending. Look closely, and you'll soon see his favorite number, 44, printed on the back of kids' soccer jerseys, in honor of the Sisks' eight years of coaching with South Valley Athletics. And then, of course, there's the family—wife Stacie, daughters Marissa Sisk, Haley Sisk and Alex Henderson and son Thomas Fotta—who will forever remember the man they affectionately called "Superdad."

Friends and family bore witness to Sisk's influence and caring during a memorial service Saturday at Eugene Faith Center. Afterward, Stacie Sisk spoke of a man who made himself memorable, even to his most casual acquaintances.

"He made an imprint on you," she said, "even if he just met you. There was something so distinct about him that always left an impression."

Sisk said she and her husband "crammed so many memory-making moments" into their marriage, that it was as if they had been married 20 years.

"He was that way with everything," she said. "The most important person in the world was the one standing in front of him at that very moment. When you're with him, it's all about you. I hope I can continue to be the kind of person he showed everybody how to be. I want to give that kind of love."

Sisk said her husband's talents shone clearly through his work in advertising and production.

"He would take a commercial or a logo and just make it come alive," she said. "He would take nothing and make it something. That's the way he was in life. He would take driving to McDonald's for a Filet-o-

Fish and make it a meaningful, impactful experience."

Hank Sisk's enthusiasm rubbed off on at least one youth, who came to him with the notion to make films of his own. When 18-year old Justin Crowe graduated from high school, Sisk gave him his old computer, which he used for film editing and contained sophisticated software, to Crowe as a graduation present. Crowe took his talents to the University of Oregon. His latest production—a video that played at Sisk's memorial service.

Stacie Sisk has yet to return to work at Cottage Grove's Wells Fargo Bank. She says the couple's house is quiet now, with just her and her 16-year old daughter there.

"We're giving it our best shot," she said. "We love this community. I'm looking forward to going back to the bank. It's been amazing to get to know customers and business owners. One customer even found out her husband had the same type of cancer Hank did. We're still friends with her. As ill as he was, Hank called to encourage her husband."

Sisk said her family hopes to stay in Cottage Grove.

"We hope to keep our home and memories here," she said. "It's important to the kids. We want to remember a great husband, father, and friend. He loved superheroes and became one. He was an awesome man."

Couple Battles Cancer Together

Byline: Mark Baker The Register-Guard

See them walk hand-in-hand. See the way they look at each other, the way they touch each other.

They say all you need is love, and nothing could be more true for Hank and Stacie Sisk of Cottage Grove.

"A hugely amount," says Hank Sisk, a 40-year-old producer of television commercials in Eugene, when asked if the strength he gathers from his 20-month marriage to Stacie has helped him fight his gastrointestinal cancer. Doctors estimated he had six months to live when his cancer was diagnosed in 2003.

"They say that if you're happy, you're healthier," says Stacie Sisk, whose breast cancer was diagnosed in January.

What are the odds that a man and a woman would fall in love in their 30s, while he was battling an extremely rare form of cancer, not knowing how much time they'd have together, and then she would develop cancer herself?

Doctors at the Willamette Valley Cancer Center in Springfield, where both Hank and Stacie receive their chemotherapy treatments in the same chair, say they've never seen such a thing before, Hank Sisk says. They've seen fathers and sons diagnosed around the same time, brothers, sisters, etc. But not this, not a new bride and groom in the prime of their lives.

So who better to serve as ambassadors for the 15th annual American Cancer Society's Relay for Life of Eugene-Springfield that begins at noon today at Lane Community College and goes until noon Saturday?

"It all just kind of fell into place," Stacie Sisk says. "This is where we are, this is what we're supposed to do."

The event began in Tacoma in 1985 and is now held in thousands of cities across America, and in others around the world, to raise money to find a cure for cancer and for educational programs and prevention. The Eugene-Springfield event began in 1992 at the University of Oregon and moved in 2003 to LCC, where organizers say it has grown into one of the most successful cancer relays on the West Coast.

"And that's just incredible," says Marc Toy, a spokesman for the Eugene office of the American Cancer Society. "You're talking about beating out cities like Portland and Seattle."

While that first Eugene event raised $11,028, last year's relay collected $530,000. This year's goal is $555,000. The total raised during the past 14 events in Eugene is $3,144,991, according to figures provided by the American Cancer Society. About 175 teams, many consisting of employees from area businesses, are registered for this year's relay.

"This is one disease that affects everybody," says Jeanne Havercroft, who started the Eugene Relay for Life in 1992 with her friend Mary Hudzikiewicz, past president of the Eugene chapter of the ACS. Two years later, Havercroft was found to have breast cancer herself.

"(This event) is going to go on and on, and I don't think people thought it would go 10 years," says Havercroft, whose husband, Bob Havercroft, died of cancer in 1994, the same year Jeanne's cancer was diagnosed.

The Sisks have never participated in the relay before. Stacie Sisk, who works for Eugene mortgage broker The Lending Team, already has had four surgeries to remove her cancer. She was at a networking meeting for area businesswomen this spring when a business partner introduced her to the group and talked of her brave fight against breast cancer. Also at the meeting was someone from the Eugene ACS office.

One thing led to another and Tinker Flom, community relationship manager for the ACS in Eugene, invited Stacie and Hank to be this year's ambassadors at the Relay for Life and share their powerful story.

"We wanted to help people, that's the biggest thing," says Hank, who has appendiatic cancer - so rare he's only heard of three others in Oregon who have it - three years ago.

Hank and Stacie, who have been friends for 10 years but did not start dating until both became divorced, have three daughters - Alex, 12, Marissa, 6, and Haley, 4 - from their first marriages. The children will walk with them at the relay, assuming Stacie is able to do so.

She's scheduled to undergo her fifth chemotherapy treatment today.

"We're hoping the reaction she has isn't so severe that she can't come out," Hank Sisk says.

Hank's cancer was so prevalent throughout his abdomen a couple of years ago that he could not find a surgeon willing to operate. That is until a friend's wife, a surgical nurse, recommended Dr. David DeHaas of Eugene.

DeHaas told Hank, who was then wearing a morphine patch 24 hours a day because of the pain, that surgery would be risky, but he thought he could remove much of the cancer that was causing the pain and "stabilize" it.

DeHaas removed five pounds of cancerous tissue from Hank's abdomen.

"I am so fortunate to be alive...' Hank says.

And to be in love.

AMERICAN CANCER SOCIETY RELAY FOR LIFE

What: 15th annual 24-hour fund-raiser for medical research, celebration of cancer survivors and a commemoration

This was written by our Pastor:

Hank and Stacie Sisk. This morning, we are going to hear an amazing story of love, courage, and hope. Hank and Stacie Sisk have already lived two or three lifetimes. We met Hank after our youth helped him get his Christmas decorations up. He had been diagnosed with an aggressive form of cancer. We later learned that while he was in remission, his wife was herself diagnosed with breast cancer. He saw her through that terrible ordeal and things began to look hopeful again. Once she was pronounced cancer-free, in a cruel twist of fate, Hank's cancer returned.

Now at this point, no one would blame these folks if they got depressed and withdrawn. Instead, they began a film project (Hank is a producer). The film, "The Letter," is a short story of God's faithfulness to a family whose daughter has cancer. Word of their story made the local news. Oprah Winfrey expressed interest in interviewing them.

His passion was to get the word out that cancer can be beaten and that those facing such a diagnosis have reason for hope. Their story has reached not only Oregon but the whole country. Here is what I'd like to do. There has been a fund set up to help this amazing family financially. Just ask at the Cottage Grove (Oregon) Wells Fargo Bank about the Hank Sisk Fund.

If you want to give something through our Church, just mark an envelope with their names, and mail to: Cottage Grove Faith Center Cottage Grove, OR 97424

We'll see that they get it. For those of you lucky enough to be attending our church today, let's sit back and hear a mighty story of the grace of God expressed through two amazing people. -Pastor Jim September 28, 2008

Made in the USA
Middletown, DE
03 May 2019